proActive

Yoga

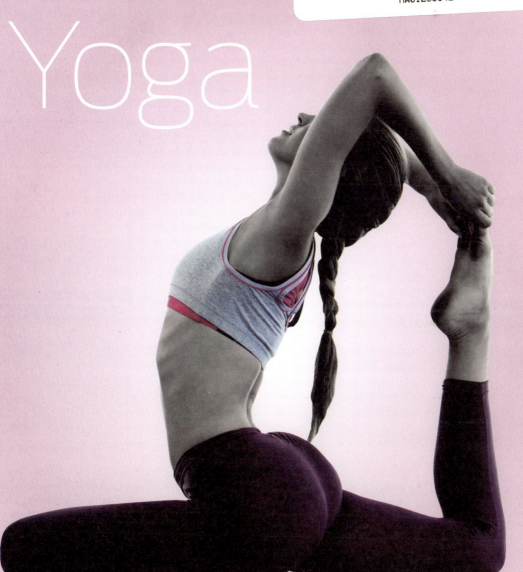

proActive

Yoga

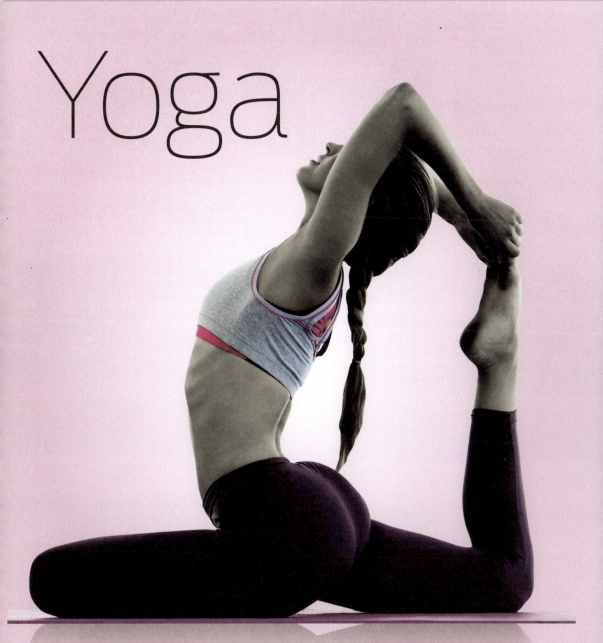

Goldie Karpel Oren

hinkler

Published by Hinkler Pty Ltd 2022
45–55 Fairchild Street
Heatherton Victoria 3202 Australia
www.hinkler.com.au

hinkler

Copyright © Hinkler Pty Ltd 2013, 2020, 2022

Created by Moseley Road Inc.
Editorial Director: Lisa Purcell
Art Director: Brian MacMullen
Photographer: Jonathan Conklin Photography, Inc.
Editor: Erica Gordon-Mallin
Designers: Danielle Scaramuzzo, Patrick Johnson
Author: Goldie Karpel Oren
Model: Lana Russo
Nutrition writer: Cori D. Cohen, RD
Illustrator: Hector Aiza/3DLabz Animation India
Cover Design: Sam Grimmer

All rights reserved. No part of this publication may be reproduced, stored in a retrieval system, or transmitted in any way or by any means, electronic, mechanical, photocopying, recording or otherwise, without the prior written permission of Hinkler Pty Ltd.

ISBN: 978 1 4889 4653 0

Printed and bound in China

Always do the warm-up exercises before attempting any individual exercises. It is recommended that you check with your doctor or healthcare professional before commencing any exercise regime. While every care has been taken in the preparation of this material, the publishers and their respective employees or agents will not accept responsibility for injury or damage occasioned to any person as a result of participation in the activities described in this book.

Contents

What is yoga?..8
Home practice..10
Breath control..14
Yoga and nutrition..18
Full-body anatomy..22

STANDING POSES..24
Mountain Pose..26
Upward Salute..28
Warrior II...30
Extended Triangle Pose..32
Extended Side Angle Pose..34
Half Moon Pose..36
Warrior I..38
Revolved Triangle Pose..40
Revolved Extended Side Angle Pose...............................42
Warrior III..44
Revolved Half Moon Pose...46
Garland Pose..48
Chair Pose..50
Twisting Chair Pose..51
Low Lunge..52
High Lunge..54
Standing Split Pose..56
Tree Pose...58
Eagle Pose...60
Extended Hand-to-Big-Toe Pose.....................................62
Lord of the Dance Pose..64

STANDING FORWARD BENDS....................................66
Cat Pose..68
Intense Side Stretch..70
Standing Half Forward Bend to Standing Forward Bend.....72
Wide-Legged Forward Bend..74

BACKBENDS ... 76
Cow Pose ... 78
Upward-Facing Dog ... 80
Cobra Pose ... 82
Locust Pose ... 84
Half-Frog Pose ... 86
Bow Pose ... 88
Bridge Pose ... 90
Wheel Pose ... 92
Camel Pose ... 94
Fish Pose ... 96
Pigeon Pose ... 98

ARM SUPPORTS ... 100
Plank Pose ... 102
Chaturanga ... 104
Side Plank ... 106
Crow Pose ... 108
Side Crow Pose ... 110
Eight-Angle Pose ... 112

INVERTED POSES ... 114
Downward-Facing Dog ... 116
Plow Pose ... 118
Shoulder Stand ... 120
Head Stand ... 122

SEATED & SEATED TWIST POSES ... 124
Staff Pose ... 126
Easy Pose ... 128
Hero Pose ... 130
Cow-Face Pose ... 132
Full Lotus Pose ... 134
Full Boat Pose ... 136

Sage's Pose ... 138
Half Lord of the Fishes Pose ... 140
Monkey Pose ... 142

SEATED FORWARD BENDS ... 144
Child's Pose ... 146
Extended Puppy Pose ... 148
Bound Angle Pose ... 150
Fire Log Pose ... 152
Head-to-Knee Forward Bend ... 154
Revolved Head-to-Knee Pose ... 156
Seated Forward Bend ... 158
Wide-Angle Seated Forward Bend ... 160

RECLINING POSES ... 162
Knees-to-Chest Pose ... 164
Reclining Big Toe Pose ... 166
Reclining Twist ... 168
Corpse Pose ... 170

YOGA FLOWS ... 172
Sun Salutation A ... 174
Sun Salutation B ... 174
Hip-Opening Flow ... 176
Well-Rounded Flow ... 176
Hamstrings Flow ... 178
Twisting Flow ... 178
Intermediate Flow ... 180
Advanced Flow ... 180

Conclusion ... 183
Glossary ... 184
Icon Index ... 188
About the Author/Credits ... 192

What is yoga?

The practice of yoga not only disciplines your body, but it also helps you discipline your mind

Yoga has been practiced since ancient times. These days, when we hear the word *yoga* we think of a physical exercise of stretching and relaxing. Yet, the physical practice is just one aspect of yoga.

The mind-body connection

Yoga is more than just another form of fitness: the discipline transcends the physicality of its postures. Yoga is also a mental and spiritual practice, in the sense that the work that goes into aligning your body can also be used to align your mind. In yoga, we are trying to calm our mental fluctuations. Our minds have a tendency to think in the past and in the future; so, while our bodies are in the present moment, we have to practice keeping our minds and thoughts in the present, too. You will find, by practicing this technique, that you are more fully present on a daily basis.

The word *yoga* means to "yoke" or to "unite," and the discipline aims to bring the mind and body into sync with each other. This is accomplished through the three main components of yoga: breathing, postures, and meditation. It is thought that through the physical practice of doing poses and breathing the yoga student is enabled to then sit and meditate, allowing the mind and body to become "one."

The most tangible parts of yoga are the asanas, or postures, of which there are hundreds. Of great importance is also Pranayama, or breath control (see box below). As a student of yoga, it is through the physical effort of attaining the postures and controlling your breath that you learn to focus and calm your mind as you fully immerse yourself in your practice.

Putting asanas together

This book contains a well-balanced selection of asanas. By performing these poses and learning how to put them together to form seamless flows, you will build strength and flexibility while improving your concentration and willpower. You will learn to control your body with your mind and come to understand that, as in life, with time and patience you can overcome many obstacles.

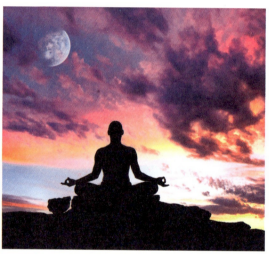

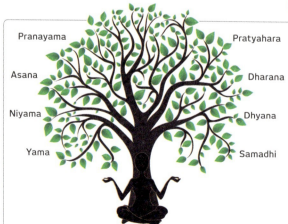

The eight limbs of yoga
One of the most famous yogic texts is the *Yoga Sutras*. This classic book, compiled by the second-century-BC scholar Patanjali, states the guidelines for yoga practice, including the eight-limbed path a yoga student should follow. According to Patanjali, the eight limbs of yoga are:

1. Yama (abstinence)
2. Niyama (observance)
3. Asana (posture)
4. Pranayama (breath control)
5. Pratyahara (sense withdrawal)
6. Dharana (concentration)
7. Dhyana (meditation)
8. Samadhi (contemplation, absorption, or superconscious state)

WHAT IS YOGA?

Challenge yourself
Your breath will get you through your poses—even the ones you find most demanding. For instance, challenge yourself to hold Camel Pose (see pages 94–95) for 30 seconds to a minute, which is about 5 to 10 long, deep breath cycles. Not only will you stretch the entire front of your body, you will also cultivate internal strength, stamina, and willpower. Stay in the position longer than you want to. Finding stillness of the body and stillness of the mind is the most challenging aspect of yoga. Holding the poses is often more difficult than moving and flowing.

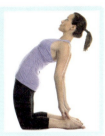

You're stronger than you think
As you tackle new asanas, you will find that your mind often tells you to give up before your body really needs to come out of a pose. Ignore that voice: while practicing yoga you must learn to distinguish between discomfort and pain. If you do suffer actual pain from an injury then come out of a pose; otherwise, try to breathe through any discomfort.

At times you will have intense sensations in your muscles—it is normal to have these feelings while holding a yoga pose. Yet sometimes you have to disregard what your mind is telling you and move beyond thinking, "I can't hold this any longer." Your body is strong enough to hold the posture for longer than you think. By holding a yoga pose for a few extra breaths, you will begin to build inner strength. You will learn that you are stronger than you imagined.

Get healthier with yoga
Yoga carries many physical and emotional health benefits. By practicing yoga, you can improve your posture, balance, flexibility, and strength. You will build stamina and endurance while toning your muscles. Yoga helps with back pain and arthritis by lubricating the joints.

Yoga has been known to improve such all-too-common ailments as poor digestion, asthma, depression, osteoporosis, high blood pressure, and other chronic medical conditions, as well as aid injury recovery.

Practicing yoga can help to raise your metabolism, increase your willpower, and heighten your body awareness, which will help you maintain a healthy weight. You may notice that by doing yoga and focusing your breath, you also build more self-awareness, have greater self-control, and feel a stronger mind-body connection.

Take a deep breath . . .
These days, we are accustomed to instant gratification—who has patience anymore? By practicing yoga and holding the poses—which can be uncomfortable—you will build patience: you will find that you can take a step back, pause, and breathe. You will discover that turning off the phone for an hour and rolling out your mat can be quite rewarding. You will realize, when you finish your practice, that you can take a guilt-free hour to shut out your to-do lists and other distracting thoughts, following through on an important decision to focus on your breath and the alignment of your body.

You will be able to use lessons learned on the yoga mat in your daily life, knowing that no challenging situation will last forever, just as no yoga posture lasts forever. Yoga teaches you to stay completely present in every moment of your life, whether it is a good time or a bad one. We often bring stress on ourselves by worrying about the future, or by dwelling on events in the past. The thoughts in your head may actually cause the stressful time—the moment you are in may not really be all that stressful.

By changing how you think about things you can change your outlook. So give yourself an extra moment to pause and take a deep breath.

Home practice

Designating a particular area within your home as your yoga space will help you keep your focus during your yoga sessions. This is where you should practice on a regular schedule.

There is much you can learn from a competent teacher, but yoga is also well suited to solo exploration. For some, finding classes that work with their schedules may be impossible, while for others, working out with groups is intimidating. Always keep in mind, though, that whether you choose to study under a teacher in a group class or practice on your own using this book as a guide, yoga is an intensely personal discipline.

Make the world go away
The greatest challenge of practicing yoga on your own at home, rather than at a studio, lies in learning to shut out all the potential distractions. Your phone, computer, television, and family can prevent you from concentrating. When practicing at home you therefore need to create a space in which you can block out those distractions. Designate a room or area where you will always practice. Make a schedule for yourself, setting aside perhaps 15 to 30 minutes at the same time every day, five days a week. The great thing about yoga is that you don't need a lot of space—just the length of the yoga mat. When traveling, you can pack your mat in your suitcase and roll it out wherever you are.

Equipment
Yoga calls for very little equipment—just take at look at the increasingly popular outdoor yoga classes conducted in many parks. Students have little more than a towel and yoga mat, and sometimes participants perform directly on a grassy surface with no equipment at all.

To begin your home practice, you need only a cushioned surface on which to work. A thick towel, blanket, or rug will serve the purpose of protecting your back and joints during many seated and reclining poses, but purchasing a yoga mat is wise decision—especially for standing and inverted poses that require you to shift your feet or hands. Relatively inexpensive, it is quite different from a Pilates mat or a padded gym mat. A mat designed specifically

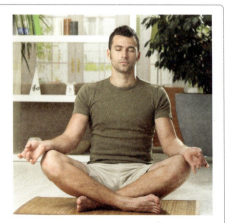

Dedicated space
There's no need to call in a carpenter to build you a home yoga studio. Your goal is to simply reserve a quiet space within your home—a space in which to retreat regularly to practice yoga.

If you live in a large house or apartment, you may have the luxury of transforming an entire room into a private yoga studio. For those in smaller spaces, you can still create a peaceful sanctuary. Just designate an area large enough for you to fully stretch and lunge freely, without obstructions. A movable screen, such as a folding Shoji screen, can lend you privacy, as can curtains or drapery that you can easily open and close.

Store your yoga mat, blocks, straps, and other gear within this space for easy access, and don't forget the atmosphere-setting extras. Gather objects that inspire you: plants, stones, and other natural objects can set the mood. A swirling image that you can meditate on or a flickering candle for your eyes to lock onto while you hold that pose just a few breaths longer can add to your yoga practice.

HOME PRACTICE

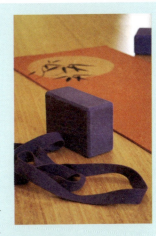

Using your tools
Think of your yoga props as tools to help you deepen your poses. Don't think that using the block and strap "makes you a beginner," or that you're not really doing the pose if you use them. In Extended Triangle Pose (see pages 32–33), for example, the point of the pose is not to reach your palms to the floor; the point of the pose is to elongate your spine, finding length on all four sides of your torso. If your hand is on the floor but your side is crunched and you can't breathe, then you're not doing yoga—you are just contorting your body. Use your block to your advantage, and create the space you need to deepen your breath.

for yoga is thin and sticky, so that you have traction to grip the floor with your hands and feet.

Using nothing more than your mat, you can perform any of the poses in this book, but adding equipment like a block or a strap will add variety to your practice. As you will see in the step-by-step portion of this book, both of these accessories also help beginners achieve postures they might not otherwise attain. They also help more advanced practitioners improve their alignment and balance.

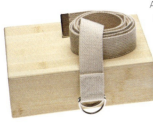

A yoga block is just that: a small brick-shaped rectangle, usually made from lightweight foam rubber or cork. These bricks extend your stretch, so place a block under your hands to find balance in poses that call for you to reach toward the floor, such as you do when performing Half Moon Pose (see pages 36–37). Blocks will also safely stretch your back or inner thighs when your sit or lie on them. Try a folded blanket if you don't have a yoga block.

Blankets make useful props, too. They cushion your back in reclining poses and raise your hips above your knees in seated poses. And best of all, you probably already have a few blankets around the house.

A yoga strap also extends your reach and enables you to hold poses longer. In poses such as Seated Forward Bend (see pages 158–159) they assist you when you need to hold onto your feet but cannot reach them. Straps also assist you if your hands do not reach each other in poses such as Cow-Face Pose (see pages 132–133).

Most yoga straps are simple affairs, made of cotton with D-rings to fasten them around your feet or hands, if necessary. Measuring from 6 to 10 feet (1.8–3 m), they are longer than regular belts, but a regular belt or long scarf can, in some cases, substitute for a yoga strap.

Clothing
During your yoga session, you want to focus on your movements and your breath—not on whether your too-snug waistband is digging into your stomach as you fold over in

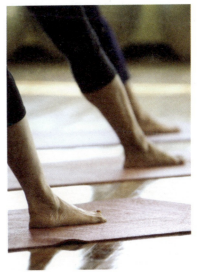

Wide-Legged Forward Bend (see pages 74–75) or if your too-loose shirt is flapping over your face when you try a Shoulder Stand (see pages 120–121). These days, there are so many choices for yoga gear, but the key factor is ease of movement—look for comfortable, form-fitting (but not tight) tops and pants, ones that do not restrict or interfere with your movement. Layering is also a good idea; for instance, wear a long-sleeved hoodie over a tank top for your warm-up session, and then shed it as your core temperature rises during your practice. You can always slip it back on during your cool-down poses.

Yoga calls for no special foot gear—in fact, leave off the socks and shoes. Practicing in bare feet will help you ground your hands and feet into the floor.

ANATOMY OF FITNESS • YOGA

Using your yoga guide
The following chapters will guide you through a wide variety of asanas. Each asana is listed under both its English name and the traditional Sanskrit name, where applicable. For all of the asanas, you'll find a short overview of the pose, photos with step-by-step instructions demonstrating how to do it, some tips on how to perform it, and anatomical illustrations that highlight key muscles. Some asanas have accompanying variations, shown in the modification box.

Alongside each exercise is a quick-read panel that features an at-a-glance illustration of the targeted areas, an estimate of the level of difficulty, and the average amount of time you'll need to complete the exercise. For yoga, "duration" is measured in breaths—in other words, the minimum number of inhalations and exhalations you should take while holding the pose. The last category is a caution list: if you have one of the issues listed, it is best to avoid that pose.

Following the step-by step chapters is a selection of sample flows. These sequences include the classic Sun Salutations, as well as flows that target specific areas, such as the hips, hamstrings, or core, and flows that offer full-body focus. You can make your practice your own by going at your own pace; if you like, you can stay in the listed poses longer than recommended, taking extra breaths whenever you need to.

Beginnings and endings
To begin most yoga sessions, take a seated posture, and close your eyes. Use this time to center yourself and bring your awareness to your breath.

From the seated position you can rise to move through the poses in the sample flows, or you can craft your own flows as you begin to master some of the asanas. You will note that the end positions of certain poses are listed as the starting poses of others—some poses just naturally segue into others. As you learn the poses, you will begin to see how they work together to

Terms to know
Certain terms that are often heard in a yoga class will appear throughout the book.

energy up: Energy isn't tangible, but in the yoga practice you are moving stale energy around and trying to lift your energy levels. "Energy up" is a subtle feeling of an upward lift.

vinyasa: The Sanskrit word *vinyasa* literally means "to link or connect." In yoga, vinyasa can also mean a specific sequence of breath-synchronized movements used to transition between sustained postures: for example, you can perform the sequence of Plank Pose, Chaturanga, Upward-Facing Dog, Downward-Facing Dog as a transition between poses, or practice it between the right and left sides. Vinyasa yoga is also known as "flow yoga," and the name is an apt one: when performed properly one pose should run together in a seamless flow of movement and breath.

alignment: In the yoga practice each pose has an ideal position of the body. If the body is in alignment, then it is placed in a proper way so that the muscles can work more effectively; they don't have to grip or struggle to hold the position, thus preventing injury. Each pose has its own alignment points, such as where to place the hands, feet, or torso, so learning a pose means also learning its proper points of alignment.

heel-to-heel alignment: When the feet are separated wide apart, if you were to draw a line from one foot to the other the heels would be on the same line. This type of alignment is used when practicing internally rotated postures.

heel-to-arch alignment: When the feet are separated wide apart, if you were to draw a line from the front foot it would intersect with the inner arch of the back foot. This type of alignment is used in externally rotated postures.

internally rotate: The body part moves in toward the center of the body.

externally rotate: The body part moves away from the center of the body.

ground down: To press the hands or feet (foundation) into the floor.

HOME PRACTICE

Yoga hand positions

In yoga, how you hold your hands is often part of a pose. These hand positions, called *mudras*, are said to have a reflex reaction in a specific part of the brain. Taking a particular hand position is then thought to direct energy flow to that part. Some of the most common mudras are:

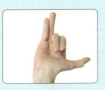

Vishnu Mudra: Curl your index and middle fingers downward, while keeping your ring and pinky fingers close together and pointed outward. Use this mudra while practicing the breathing technique Anuloma Viloma (see page 16).

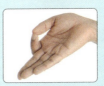

Gyan Mudra: Place together the tips of the index finger and thumb. This position represents knowledge and expansion.

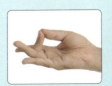

Shuni Mudra: Place together the tips of the middle finger and thumb. This position represents patience and discernment.

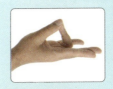

Surya Ravi Mudra. Place together the tips of your ring finger and thumb. This position represents courage and responsibility.

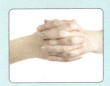

Venus Lock: Interlace the fingers of both hands, with the right pinky down for women, and the left pinky down for men. This mudra represents sensuality and sexuality.

Prayer Mudra: Place the palms of both hands together. This position, which you assume before starting a yoga flow, is said to balance the positive (male) and negative (female) sides of the body.

form seamless flows. And "flow" itself is the goal: a flowing sequence focuses the mind and synchronizes it with the body and breath, thereby drawing you deeper into the practice. Try to move smoothly from pose to pose, using your breath to help move you.

After you have completed your practice, you can then begin to cool down and calm your brain with several stretches and forward bends to prepare for your final deep relaxation, called Corpse Pose, or Savasana (see pages 170–171).

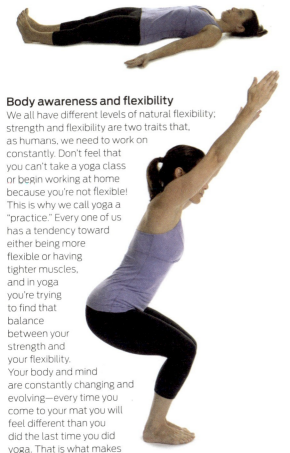

Body awareness and flexibility

We all have different levels of natural flexibility; strength and flexibility are two traits that, as humans, we need to work on constantly. Don't feel that you can't take a yoga class or begin working at home because you're not flexible! This is why we call yoga a "practice." Every one of us has a tendency toward either being more flexible or having tighter muscles, and in yoga you're trying to find that balance between your strength and your flexibility. Your body and mind are constantly changing and evolving—every time you come to your mat you will feel different than you did the last time you did yoga. That is what makes the yoga practice interesting. You may do the same poses time and time again, and yet each time you'll find something new to work on. An advanced practitioner is not necessarily someone who can come into the most challenging pose; being advanced is having the body awareness and control to work the subtleties of each pose.

Breath control

In yoga, although much emphasis is placed on the physical movement of the limbs and body, another kind of physical action is just as important: the breath.

Just about all of us take breathing for granted; after all, breathing is essential to life—it's not something we need to think about in order to do. Yet, to truly benefit from your yoga practice, you must first learn to breathe properly. Your breath will guide you through your practice.

Connecting breath and movement

The style of the sample sequences found at the end of this book is that of a "vinyasa flow." The Sanskrit term *vinyasa* means "to link or connect." In your practice, you are linking your breath with your movement, and your movement with your breath. You will begin to create a moving meditation.

After you have learned the poses and begin to perform them regularly, you will learn to hold them and then flow from one to the next. Because you'll focus on lengthening and deepening your breath, you will soon find that yoga is simply a breathing exercise. If you find yourself holding your breath or breathing heavily, take a step back and reevaluate your position. This may mean holding the pose for less time, choosing a less challenging variation of the posture, or resting in Child's Pose (see pages 146–147).

Focusing on the present moment

If you are like most people, your mind constantly jumps from thought to thought, lingering on situations and stories from your past and planning your future, so that much of the time you forget to live in the present moment. Your breath is the tool that can anchor you to the present moment. By concentrating on your breath, you force yourself to put aside any other thoughts that may be filling up your brain.

When it is deep and mindful, your breath will help to calm your nervous system. This kind of breath will help reduce stress by stimulating the parasympathetic response of the central nervous system, instead of the fight-or-flight response, which increases adrenaline. This relaxation response will help to quiet your mind, reduce stress, and make you feel good when you leave your mat.

Pranayama

Pranayama, or the science of yoga breathing, is the fourth limb of the discipline of yoga (see page 8) and the first principle on which anyone beginning a yoga practice should concentrate. Learning to breathe properly is essential.

In Sanskrit, *prana* means "life-force energy," and *ayama* means "to control or extend." Together they form the word *pranayama*, which means "extension of the life force," or "breath control." The practice of yoga calls for us to pay close attention to the process of breathing in and out that we usually take for granted.

Practicing Ujjayi, the Ocean Breath

Don't be put off by the loud sound of your breath when practicing this technique. You know you are performing it correctly when you hear a hissing sound in the back of your throat. To begin your practice, sit up tall in a comfortable position, and assume Easy Pose (see pages 128–129).

1. Place your hand in front of your mouth, and imagine that it is a mirror. Open your mouth, and exhale a *hah* sound as if you were fogging up the mirror. That breath comes from the back of the throat.

2. Now close your mouth, and try to breathe in a similar way, as if you were again fogging up that imaginary mirror. You will notice a hissing sound coming from the back of your throat. This is the beginning of practicing the Ujjayi breathing technique.

3. Complete about 8 to 10 breath cycles, inhaling and exhaling with this slight constriction in the back of your throat.

As you begin to feel more comfortable using this type of breathing technique you will naturally start to breathe in this way throughout the entire vinyasa yoga practice. The Ujjayi breath will start to flow from one breath to the next and will help you to connect your movement with your breathing.

Ujjayi Pranayama

There are several ways to manipulate the breath. One of the most common is Ujjayi Pranayama. This breathing technique calms the brain and creates internal heat.

When done correctly, Ujjayi sounds like the ocean, hence it is often called Ocean Breath. During the execution of Ujjayi Pranayama, the mouth stays closed, and there is a slight constriction of the throat as you inhale and exhale. Throughout the entire asana practice, try to match the length of your inhales with your exhales so that your breath is seamless. You can begin by lengthening your breath to a count of 4, inhaling on a count of 4, and exhaling on a count of 4. You can then lengthen your inhalation and your exhalation to a count of 5 or 6.

Dirga Pranayama

Dirga Pranayama is a three-part breathing technique that demonstrates how to fully fill your lungs and then exhale completely. It is great breathing technique for beginners, and it is also one that all of us can use in times of stress. When you feel overwhelmed by stress or fear, you begin to breathe rapidly and shallowly; Dirga Pranayama can help you remain calm by slowing down your breath and allowing you to focus more clearly.

To practice Dirga Pranayama, you can begin in a sitting posture, but to get the most calming effect, lie in Corpse Pose (see pages 170–171) and close your eyes, letting your body and facial muscles fully relax. Concentrate for a moment on the natural rhythm of your inhalations and exhalations.

1. Inhale deeply through your nose, filling your chest cavity, so that your belly expands for a count of 2, and pause for a moment.

2. Continue to expand your belly as you fill the next third of your lungs to another count of 2.

3. Continue to expand your belly as you fill the final third of your lungs to another count of 2, pause, and then exhale as smoothly as you can for a count of 6. Repeat to 5 times before beginning a yoga session.

Kapalabhati

Kapal means "skull," and *bhati* means "shining"; together the two words mean "shining skull." This is a breathing technique that will cleanse your sinuses. In Kapalabhati,

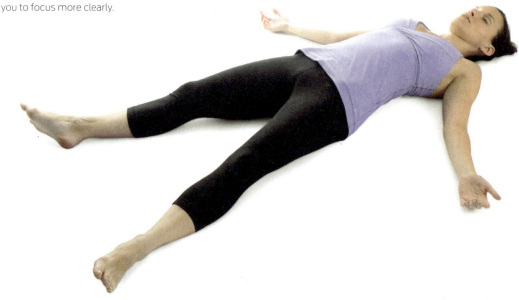

BREATH CONTROL

you control your breath by sharply exhaling while pumping your abdominal muscles in and out. The inhalation is passive, while the exhalation is forceful and sharp. The sharp and rapid exhales will help your lungs to clear any waste from your air passageways.

To practice Kapalabhati, sit up tall in a comfortable position, either in Easy Pose (see pages 128–129) or Hero Pose (see pages 130–131).

1. Close your eyes and your mouth, and relax your abdominal muscles.

2. Keeping your mouth closed, breathe only through your nose. Inhale once normally, and then exhale normally.

3. Inhale halfway, and begin to exhale sharply out of your nose in short, quick breaths while contracting your abdominal muscles. Continue doing this on each exhale. Think of drawing your stomach in and up as you pump and breathe diaphragmatically. Allow your inhale to be passive so that you are only focusing on the exhale.

4. When you are finished with your cycle, exhale all of your breath. Then, inhale once normally, and then exhale. On the next inhalation, hold your breath for as long as you can comfortably hold it, and then exhale all of the breath.

Begin with 20 cycles of Kapalabhati, and then increase the number of cycles as you become more comfortable with this technique. You can repeat the entire technique 2 to 3 times.

Anuloma Viloma
By practicing Anuloma Viloma, also called Alternate Nostril Breathing, you will create more balance between your right and left nasal passageways. As humans we don't always breathe through both of our nostrils equally; there is usually one side that is more dominant. It is said that practicing Anuloma Viloma will help to purify the energetic channels of the subtle body so that *prana* (or "life-force energy") can flow through you more easily. This breathing technique will also help to calm your mind, relieve stress, and help you prepare for a seated meditation.

Sithali
The Sithali breathing technique is perfect for the end of a rigorous yoga session because it cools the body, hence its other name, Cooling Breath.

One nostril at a time
To practice Anuloma Viloma, or Alternate Nostril Breathing: sit up tall in a comfortable position, either in Easy Pose (see pages 128–129) or Hero Pose (see pages 130–131).

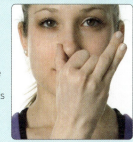

1. Lift your right hand, and bend your index and middle fingers down while keeping your thumb, ring finger, and pinky lifted. This is the Vishnu Mudra (see page 13).

2. Inhale once normally, and then exhale normally.

3. Close off your right nostril with your right thumb and inhale through your left nostril.

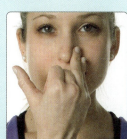

4. Use your ring finger to close off both nostrils and hold the breath.

5. Keeping your ring finger on your left nostril, exhale out of your right nostril.

6. Inhale through your right nostril, and then close off both nostrils and pause to hold the breath.

7. Exhale out of your left nostril. This is one round of Anuloma Viloma.

Continue repeating steps 2 through 8 for another 3 to 5 cycles. When you are finished practicing Anuloma Viloma you can sit quietly in a seated meditation.

Unlike nearly all other yoga breathing techniques, which call for you to breathe through your nostrils, Sithali calls for you to breathe through your mouth.

To practice Sithali, sit up tall in a comfortable position, either in Easy Pose (see pages 128–129) or Hero Pose (see pages 130–131), and take two or three deep inhales and exhales through your nose to prepare.

1. Purse your lips, and then curl your tongue, rolling the sides upward to form a tube. Stick the end of the tongue out between your pursed lips. (If you can't curl your tongue, just make a small O shape with your mouth.)

2. Inhale through the tube of your tongue.

3. Exhale through both nostrils.

4. Keeping your tongue curled, repeat 5 to 10 times until you feel the cool-down effect.

ANATOMY OF FITNESS • YOGA

Yoga and nutrition

Eating a healthful and balanced diet will help you get the most from your yoga practice. Focus on fresh, high-quality foods that boost energy without adding toxins to your body.

The connection between fitness and nutrition has long been emphasized, and for good reason. Whether you are taking up yoga to improve a health condition, de-stress, or get energized, eating the proper quantity and balance of nutrients is essential to achieving your goals. Consuming the right types and amounts of nutrients and fluid helps you to exercise for longer and at a higher intensity. It also aids in muscle recovery after workouts, improves strength, increases energy levels, helps to maintain healthy immune function, and reduces the risk of injury and heat cramps.

Fueling for fitness

Our bodies need fuel to function, and the harder we push ourselves the more fuel we require. Professional athletes and marathon runners utilize carbohydrate loading and require hundreds of excess calories to keep them performing at their peak. But for most of us, who work out less than four times a week at low to moderate intensity, it is not necessary to take these drastic measures. Instead, as you begin practicing yoga, focus on consuming small meals with plenty of fruits, vegetables, whole grains, and nuts. Look to take in a healthy combination of carbohydrates and protein with small amounts of fat and fiber. For example, try eating a nut butter sandwich on whole-wheat toast with an apple, or a serving of Greek yogurt with fruit and low-fat granola approximately three to four hours before exercising. Then, about one half hour to an hour before working out, eat a whole fruit like a banana or orange and drink a full glass of water. The proper timing and intake of these nutrients will enhance your workout and the benefits you receive from it.

After a workout, carbohydrates help to replenish muscle fuel lost during exercise, while protein aids in the repair of damaged muscle tissue and the development of new tissue. Aim to eat a meal or snack 15 to 60 minutes after engaging in physical activity. Some healthful meal suggestions include a chicken or vegetable stir-fry, whole-wheat pita with turkey, hummus, and salad, or a brown rice bowl with beans and steamed vegetables. If you are on the go and cannot prepare a healthful meal within the hour, stock your gym bag with nutritional supplements. A variety of bars on the market contain a balanced blend of carbohydrates, protein, and essential vitamins and minerals.

A little protein goes a long way

There is a common misconception that loading up on protein is the key to building muscle mass. Although protein plays an important role in the growth and repair of muscle tissue, most adults who live in developed countries already get more than enough from their typical daily diets. For adults engaging in approximately one hour of exercise three (or fewer) times a week, the daily recommendation for protein is 46 grams for females and 56 grams for males. One ounce of meat, poultry, or fish, which is similar in size to a small matchbox, contains 7 grams of protein. This means that 6.5 ounces of meat, fish, or poultry provides the average female with all of the protein she needs in a day and 8 ounces meets the daily protein requirement for most males. The portion of protein provided by one main dish at a majority of restaurants comes close to meeting these needs all on its own! Many individuals, especially those who dine out frequently, are exceeding their protein needs by more than just a few grams.

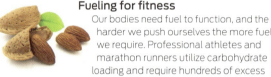

A rainbow diet

Eating the colors of the rainbow may sound like an elementary school lesson plan, but its underlying message is important for adults and children alike. Choose from a varied palette of fruits and vegetables from red berries to green spinach to violet plums—and all the shades in between. Splashing your plate with different-colored fruits and vegetables is an easy and smart way to ensure that you are getting the vitamins and minerals you need.

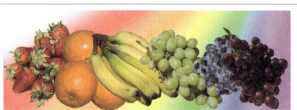

YOGA AND NUTRITION

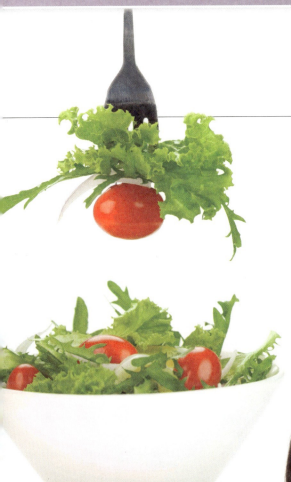

line is that you are most likely getting enough protein in your diet, but you may be getting it from the wrong foods. Choose smarter sources of protein such as tuna, salmon, chicken, turkey, nuts, and beans, and complement them with a variety of fruits and vegetables. This will not only help you to achieve your physical fitness goals, but it will also increase your energy levels and keep your heart and internal organs healthier.

Eat your veggies

What's not to like about vegetables? They are generally low-fat, low-calorie foods with a high return in vitamins and minerals—especially the green, yellow, and orange ones, which are great sources of calcium, magnesium, potassium, iron, beta-carotene, vitamin B complex, vitamin C, vitamin A, and vitamin K. As an added benefit, most vegetables contain soluble and insoluble dietary fiber.

Aim to include about 5 to 7 servings of fresh vegetables in your daily diet. Look for seasonal varieties in a rich array of colors. Choose the freshest, whole vegetables that are bright in color and feel heavy for their sizes. Whenever possible, buy small quantities that you can consume in just a day or two.

In many cases men with moderate-intensity workout regimens are consuming the same amount of protein recommended for professional athletes. Exceeding the recommended amount of protein is unnecessary and can even prove harmful.

Popular animal proteins like eggs, beef, and pork are packed with saturated fat and cholesterol. An abundance of medium- and high-fat animal proteins in the diet increases risk of heart disease and can also place unwarranted burden on the kidneys. These diets are also typically lacking in fruits and vegetables, leading to an insufficient intake of important nutrients like vitamin C, vitamin E, and folate. The bottom

ANATOMY OF FITNESS • YOGA

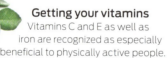

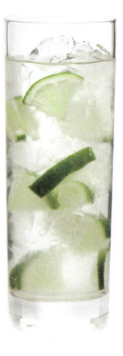

Getting your vitamins
Vitamins C and E as well as iron are recognized as especially beneficial to physically active people. Each of these nutrients contains unique properties that contribute to aerobic endurance, immune system strength, and optimal recovery from exercise. Nuts, seeds, and plant oils like sunflower oil are great sources of vitamin E, while citrus fruits, blueberries, strawberries, red peppers, and broccoli supply vitamin C. Spinach, kidney beans, and fortified grain products, such as breakfast cereals, contain iron, but our bodies are less able to absorb it from these foods than from animal sources such as meat and seafood.

Hydrate, hydrate
Consuming adequate fluid is another key factor in maximizing exercise performance and preventing injury. Proper hydration maintains optimal organ function and helps you feel your best during and after your yoga practice. It is healthy to work up a sweat while exercising; sweating is your body's way of protecting you from overheating during periods of physical exertion. When you fail to replace fluids lost through perspiration, serious issues can present. Early signs of dehydration include thirst, flushed skin, premature fatigue, increased pulse rate and breathing, and decreased exercise capacity. These symptoms can give way to dizziness and severe weakness if dehydration is allowed to persist. Most nutrition authorities recommend drinking water before, during, and after low- to moderate-intensity exercise that lasts up to an hour. For anyone exercising for more than an hour at a higher intensity, such as those who practice certain forms of "hot" yoga, it is beneficial to consume beverages that contain a combination of carbohydrates and electrolytes. A smart choice is 100 percent pure coconut water, which contains fewer calories and less sugar and sodium than many popular sports drinks. Another healthy way to replace fluids and electrolytes lost during exercise is to eat a serving of fruit or vegetables after your workout.

Control your body's destiny
Maintaining a healthy diet requires the right mind-set and a sufficient dose of determination. Life happens: we get invited to parties, suffer stressful days, and succumb to the occasional overwhelming chocolate craving. Nobody said that it was going to be as simple as waving a magic wand and never wanting French fries again! If you initiate a healthier diet by making drastic changes, it is unlikely to last; eating lettuce and broccoli for lunch and dinner Monday through Friday and then topping off a pint of chocolate fudge ice cream every weekend on "cheat days" is an inefficient and unhealthy approach to meeting your health and weight-loss goals. Starting with smart, measurable goals and staying on a realistic and positive path is the best way to achieve long-term results.

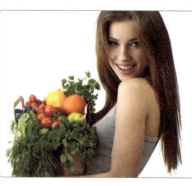

Should you go vegetarian?
Practicing yoga often brings a new and exciting awareness of your body and with it a newfound appreciation of what you consume and how it makes you feel. Maybe you start to realize that those frosted cupcakes you love are making you sluggish or the chips are causing you to bloat. Eating "clean" is a popular concept amongst yogis, athletes, and health enthusiasts alike; it means basing your diet on whole fresh foods and limiting processed foods with additives and a large list of hard-to-pronounce ingredients. Many yogis also choose to go vegetarian or vegan, eliminating animal proteins like meat, milk, and eggs from their diets. Eating a diet built upon plant proteins like legumes, nuts, and seeds can be beneficial to your heart and other organ systems, but remember that no one diet is a perfect fit for all of us. We are all unique and need to find a balance that works in our own lives and for our own bodies. If you decide to transition to a meat-free, dairy-free diet, consult with a dietitian to ensure that you are still including all of the essential vitamins and minerals that your body needs for optimal health.

Vitamins and supplements

It is always best to obtain nutrients from whole foods. If you find certain nutrient-rich foods unpalatable or they aren't readily available where you live, however, then it is crucial to take a multivitamin that contains at least 100 percent of the recommended daily value (DV) for the nutrients you need. This information can be found on the supplement package.

Find a balance that works for you. Make sure that your daily diet includes foods you enjoy so that you do not enter the weekend feeling deprived. Find healthier substitutes for the less healthful foods you crave. For example, some nutritional supplement bars deliver rich chocolate flavor to your taste buds while also providing you with 100 percent of the daily-recommended folate. They may even satisfy your sweet tooth equally as well as your favorite candy bar (which contains three times the saturated fat)!

Leading a healthier lifestyle need not mean forfeiting your social life. Dining out with friends and attending dinner parties may present more of a challenge than before, but with the right navigation tools they can be just as enjoyable. The number one rule: never arrive at a restaurant or party too hungry. Eat a whole fruit like an apple or orange and drink two glasses of water one half hour before mealtime. If you are in a rush, have your fruit and water en route to your destination. This small healthy snack will help you make better decisions and forgo nutritionally scanty starters like bread or chips and dip.

When dining out, order a healthy starter when you get to the table so that you are less tempted to pick at the contents of the bread basket. If possible, review the restaurant's offerings online beforehand to reduce the stress of finding healthy dishes on the spot. Do not be timid about asking your server to describe the contents of a sauce or how a main dish is prepared. She is there to help you and your desire to eat well is something to be proud of. Avoid fried foods and cream-based sauces such as Alfredo or vodka sauce. Instead, opt for dishes made with light olive oil or marinara sauce. If you are really craving something sweet at the end of your meal, order a dessert that everyone at the table wants to share—a great way to ensure portion control while still enjoying a sweet ending to the night.

At a dinner party, serve yourself instead of letting other people dictate what goes on your plate. When you look at your blank plate, imagine it as a diagram cut into three sections. Designate the upper left corner for starches like pasta and rice, the lower left corner for protein like turkey, chicken, or fish and the entire right side of the plate for vegetables. This will help you to retain portion control and consume a balanced meal. Do not eat quickly: scientific research has shown that it takes 20 minutes for your brain to process whether or not your stomach is full. Savor each bite and chew thoroughly to allow your brain to catch up to the state of your stomach. Once you have licked the last crumb off your plate, place your hands in your lap and make a conscious decision not to go back for seconds—at least not yet. Occupy your mind and mouth for 20 minutes by talking to friends, helping the host clear the table, or even visiting the bathroom and reciting a monologue in front of the mirror if need be! Once the 20 minutes are up you will have a better grasp on the state of your satiation. If you are still hungry, go back for the vegetable choices and drink another glass of water. Use your willpower to avoid second helpings of starch and fatty proteins like beef or pork.

Good news: you have already taken a step in the right direction by buying this fitness book and reading about better nutrition. More good news: you don't need to overhaul your life or refrigerator to achieve your goals. Initiating small changes, like substituting healthier choices for the less nutritious foods in your diet, can get you looking and feeling better as you move through your daily life.

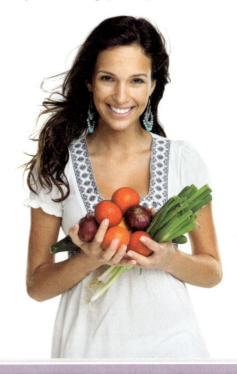

ANATOMY OF FITNESS • YOGA

Full-body anatomy

Front View

Annotation Key
* indicates deep muscles

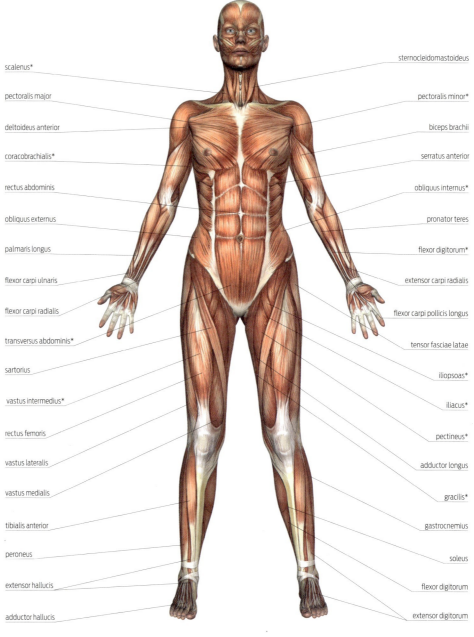

- scalenus*
- pectoralis major
- deltoideus anterior
- coracobrachialis*
- rectus abdominis
- obliquus externus
- palmaris longus
- flexor carpi ulnaris
- flexor carpi radialis
- transversus abdominis*
- sartorius
- vastus intermedius*
- rectus femoris
- vastus lateralis
- vastus medialis
- tibialis anterior
- peroneus
- extensor hallucis
- adductor hallucis

- sternocleidomastoideus
- pectoralis minor*
- biceps brachii
- serratus anterior
- obliquus internus*
- pronator teres
- flexor digitorum*
- extensor carpi radialis
- flexor carpi pollicis longus
- tensor fasciae latae
- iliopsoas*
- iliacus*
- pectineus*
- adductor longus
- gracilis*
- gastrocnemius
- soleus
- flexor digitorum
- extensor digitorum

22

FULL-BODY ANATOMY

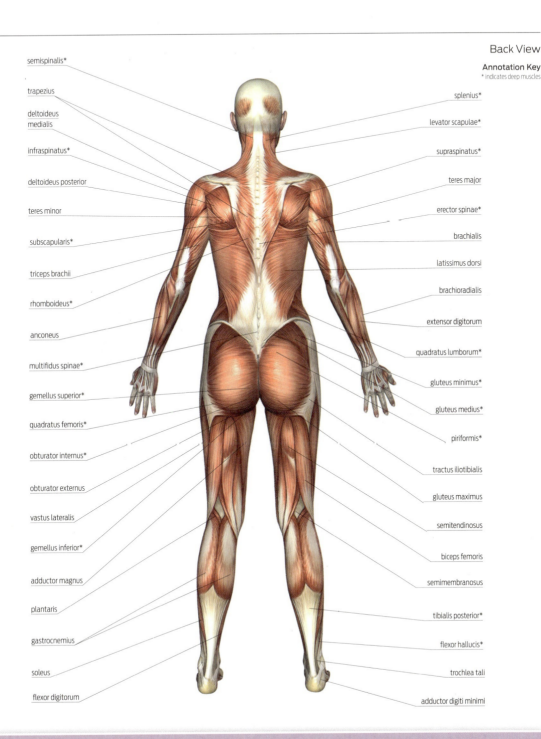

Back View

Annotation Key
* indicates deep muscles

semispinalis*
trapezius
deltoideus medialis
infraspinatus*
deltoideus posterior
teres minor
subscapularis*
triceps brachii
rhomboideus*
anconeus
multifidus spinae*
gemellus superior*
quadratus femoris*
obturator internus*
obturator externus
vastus lateralis
gemellus inferior*
adductor magnus
plantaris
gastrocnemius
soleus
flexor digitorum

splenius*
levator scapulae*
supraspinatus*
teres major
erector spinae*
brachialis
latissimus dorsi
brachioradialis
extensor digitorum
quadratus lumborum*
gluteus minimus*
gluteus medius*
piriformis*
tractus iliotibialis
gluteus maximus
semitendinosus
biceps femoris
semimembranosus
tibialis posterior*
flexor hallucis*
trochlea tali
adductor digiti minimi

23

ANATOMY OF FITNESS • YOGA

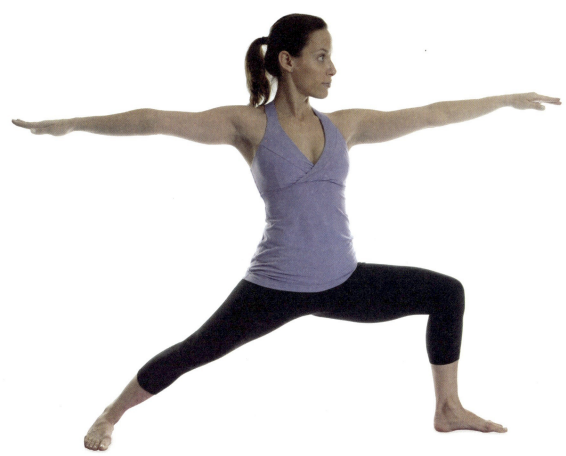

Contents

Mountain Pose 26	Garland Pose. 48
Upward Salute 28	Chair Pose. 50
Warrior II 30	Twisting Chair Pose 51
Extended Triangle Pose 32	Low Lunge 52
Extended Side Angle Pose 34	High Lunge 54
Half Moon Pose 36	Standing Split Pose 56
Warrior I 38	Tree Pose. 58
Revolved Triangle Pose. 40	Eagle Pose 60
Revolved Extended Side Angle Pose 42	Extended Hand-to-Big-Toe Pose 62
Warrior III. 44	Lord of the Dance Pose. 64
Revolved Half Moon Pose 46	

STANDING POSES

Standing Poses

Standing poses build strength and flexibility. Each pose has its own benefits, and focuses on different muscle groups. Mountain Pose is the foundation for all standing poses; within each pose, the alignment points for this pose can be found. Begin by standing in these poses for only as long as you feel comfortable. Eventually, you will be able to intensify the poses by holding them for longer periods of time.

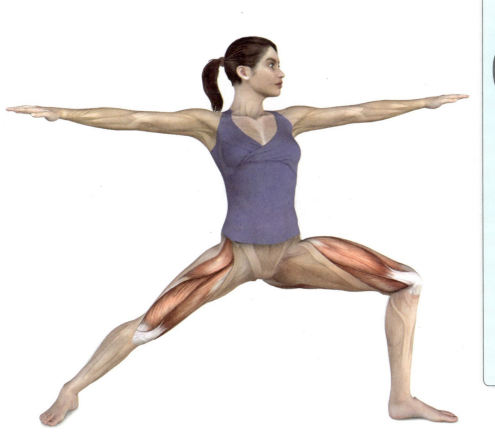

Mountain Pose

(Tadasana)

Mountain Pose forms the starting point for many standing poses. Although this posture may seem simple, it can actually be quite challenging to achieve the correct alignment.

1 Stand tall, with your feet together. Inhale, then exhale as you bring your arms to your sides.

2 Take 5 to 10 breaths as you maintain the pose. Find your balance, keeping your pelvis neutral by drawing the tip of your tailbone down toward your feet as you lift your hip bones upward. Your weight may shift in a circular motion as you balance. Root and rebound, feeling your feet grounded into the floor as you visualize energy radiating upward, from the bottom of your feet through the top of your head.

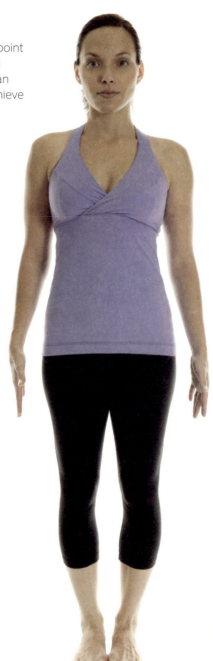

Correct form
- Release any tension in your facial area.
- Stand completely straight with shoulders stacked over hips, hips stacked over knees, and knees in line with feet.
- Visualize your pelvis as a bowl of soup—you don't want to spill it forward or backward.
- Stretch your arms straight, with energy reaching out of your fingertips.
- Keep your chin parallel to the floor, and the crown of your head pressing upward.

Avoid
- Arching your lower back.
- Pushing your ribs forward.
- Over-tucking your pelvis.
- Holding your breath.

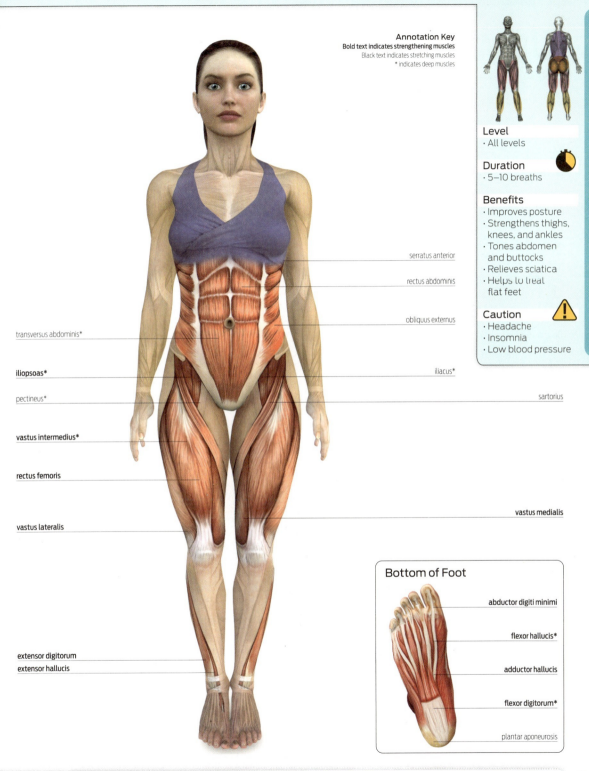

ANATOMY OF FITNESS • YOGA

Upward Salute

(Urdhva Hastasana)

Upward Salute is the second pose in the Sun Salutation A series. In the traditional posture, the arms are separated; if your shoulders are more open, you can join your hands together above your head while keeping your arms straight.

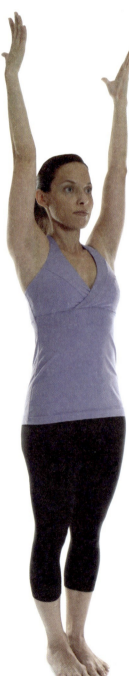

1 From Mountain Pose (pages 26–27), inhale as you reach your arms out to your sides, and continue lifting until you are standing with your arms above your head. Your hands should be shoulder-width apart.

2 Straighten your arms, and rotate your shoulders externally open so that the palms of your hands face each other, spreading up through your fingertips.

3 Gaze forward or tilt your head slightly back, and bring your gaze up to your thumbs. Hold for 1 to 5 breaths.

Upward Salute • STANDING POSES

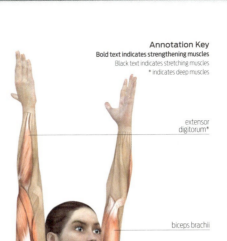

Back View

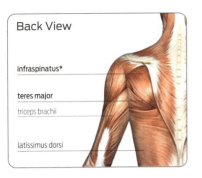

- infraspinatus*
- teres major
- triceps brachii
- latissimus dorsi

Annotation Key
Bold text indicates strengthening muscles
Black text indicates stretching muscles
* indicates deep muscles

- extensor digitorum*
- biceps brachii
- deltoideus anterior
- obliquus internus*
- obliquus externus*

- deltoideus posterior
- serratus anterior

Level
- Beginner

Duration
- 1–5 breaths

Benefits
- Stretches shoulders, arms, and belly

Caution
- Neck issues
- Shoulder issues

Correct form
- Stretch your arms completely straight from your elbows.
- Soften any tension in your shoulders.

Avoid
- Tensing your shoulders up toward your ears.
- Bending your elbows.

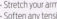

ANATOMY OF FITNESS • YOGA

Warrior II
(Virabhadrasana II)

One of the three Warrior poses performed in yoga, Warrior II often comes earlier in a sequence than Warrior I. Mastering Warrior II will help you build the inner strength and courage of a warrior.

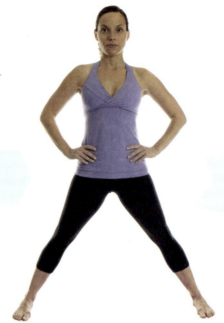

1 Stand in Mountain Pose (pages 26–27). Step or jump your feet about 3 to 4 feet apart. Turn your left foot out 90 degrees and your right foot in slightly.

2 Walk your left foot to the right several inches so that your left heel aligns with the inner arch of your right foot.

3 Keeping your left knee bent, lift your torso so that your shoulders line up over your hips. Keep a slight internal rotation to the back leg to keep your leg neutral. Extend both arms out to the sides, parallel to the floor, with palms facing downward. Continue to bend your left knee, externally rotating your left hip to open your thigh. Find a neutral pelvis. Turn your head toward the left and gaze past your fingers.

4 Hold for 1 to 5 breaths. Repeat on the other side.

Warrior II • STANDING POSES

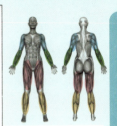

Back View

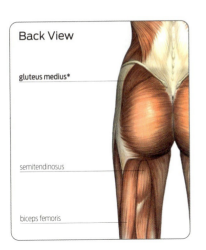

- gluteus medius*
- semitendinosus
- biceps femoris

Correct form
- Press your heels into the floor, using your inner-thigh muscles.
- Keep your shoulders directly above your hips.
- When holding the pose, make sure that your front knee is in line with your middle toe.

Avoid
- Arching your lower back.
- Leaning over your bent leg.

Annotation Key
Bold text indicates strengthening muscles
Black text indicates stretching muscles
* indicates deep muscles

Level
- Beginner/Intermediate

Duration
- 1–5 breaths

Benefits
- Strengthens thighs and arms
- Stretches shoulders, chest, and groin
- Increases stamina

Caution
- Knee issues

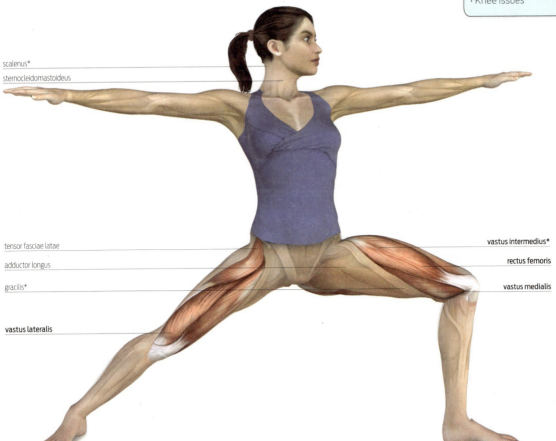

- scalenus*
- sternocleidomastoideus
- tensor fasciae latae
- adductor longus
- gracilis*
- vastus lateralis
- vastus intermedius*
- rectus femoris
- vastus medialis

ANATOMY OF FITNESS • YOGA

Extended Triangle Pose
(Utthita Trikonasana)

Extended Triangle Pose encompasses the entire body. It is a hip opener, core strengthener, side bend, twist, and heart opener.

1 Stand in Mountain Pose (pages 26–27). Step or jump your feet about 3 to 4 feet apart. Turn your left foot out 90 degrees and your right foot in slightly.

2 Walk your left foot to the right several inches so that your left heel aligns with the inner arch of your right foot.

3 Keeping both legs straight with firm thighs and your arms extended out to your sides parallel to the floor, exhale and reach your left arm and torso down to the left as you shift your hips to the right, deepening the crease in your left hip.

4 Place your left hand on your shin or on the floor on the outside of your left leg. Extend your right arm straight up, with fingers spread. Inhale as you find length across your collarbones.

5 Exhale and turn the left side of your torso toward the ceiling.

6 Inhale as you turn your head to gaze up at your right fingertips. Hold for 1 to 5 breaths. Repeat on the other side.

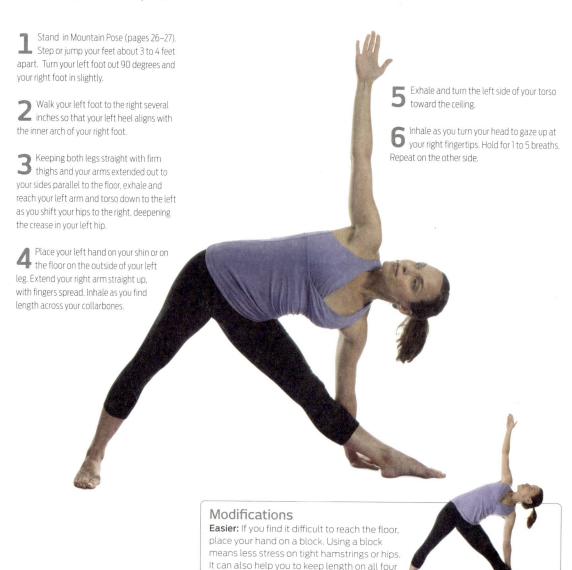

Modifications
Easier: If you find it difficult to reach the floor, place your hand on a block. Using a block means less stress on tight hamstrings or hips. It can also help you to keep length on all four sides of your torso, rather than rounding your back as you lean over.

Extended Triangle Pose • **STANDING POSES**

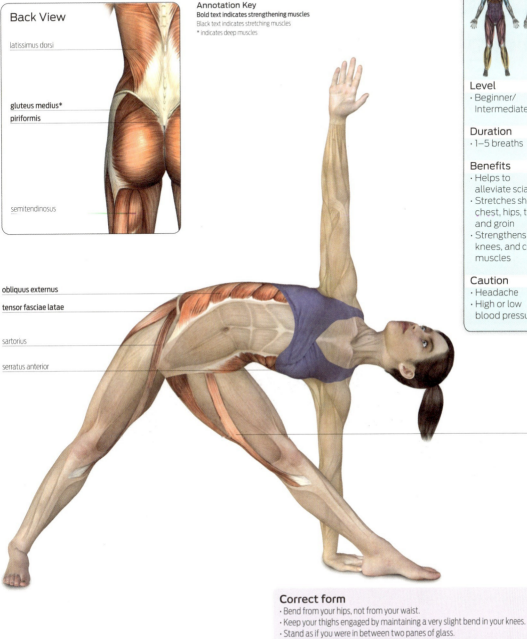

Back View

latissimus dorsi

gluteus medius*
piriformis

semitendinosus

Annotation Key
Bold text indicates strengthening muscles
Black text indicates stretching muscles
* indicates deep muscles

obliquus externus
tensor fasciae latae

sartorius
serratus anterior

gracilis

Level
- Beginner/ Intermediate

Duration
- 1–5 breaths

Benefits
- Helps to alleviate sciatica
- Stretches shoulders, chest, hips, thighs, and groin
- Strengthens ankles, knees, and core muscles

Caution
- Headache
- High or low blood pressure

Correct form
- Bend from your hips, not from your waist.
- Keep your thighs engaged by maintaining a very slight bend in your knees.
- Stand as if you were in between two panes of glass.
- If you choose to use a block, position it on the floor directly under your shoulder.

Avoid
- Locking your knees.
- Crunching the bottom side of your torso while bending.
- Leaning forward.

Extended Side Angle Pose

(Utthita Parsvakonasana)

Extended Side Angle Pose is a great stretch for the sides of your torso. When performed correctly, your upper arm, spine, and back leg should form one continuous diagonal line. You can try different variations of this pose, depending on how you feel.

1 Stand in Mountain Pose (pages 26–27). Step or jump your feet about 3 to 4 feet apart. Turn your left foot out 90 degrees and your right foot in slightly.

2 Walk your left foot to the right several inches so that your left heel aligns with the inner arch of your right foot. Extend your arms out to your sides, parallel to the floor.

3 Keeping your right leg straight, with the thigh slightly internally rotated, press weight into the pinky toe edge of your right foot. Exhale as you extend your torso to the left, reaching your left hand to the floor on the outside of your foot.

4 Inhale and extend your right arm straight up to the ceiling. Turn your right hand to face the floor, externally rotating the entire arm as you exhale and reach over your ear.

5 Inhale and lengthen your torso. Exhale and pivot the left side of your body clockwise toward the ceiling.

6 Turn your gaze underneath your right arm up toward the ceiling, and hold for 1 to 5 breaths. Repeat on the other side.

Correct form
- Press your bottom knee into your bottom arm, using that resistance to open your right hip.
- Ground your back foot into the floor.
- Keep your upper arm extended, and your back leg straight.
- Keep the knee of your bottom foot in line with your toes, pointing forward.

Avoid
- Crunching your bottom ribs.
- Allowing your shoulders to round forward.

Extended Side Angle Pose • **STANDING POSES**

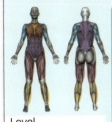

Modifications
Harder: Wrap your bottom arm under your right thigh and wrap the other arm behind your back to join your hands together.

Easier: If you find it difficult to reach the floor, place the hand of your bottom arm on a block. You can also rest your forearm on your thigh.

Level
- Intermediate

Duration
- 1–5 breaths

Benefits
- Stretches hips, groin, side of the body, and spine
- Strengthens and stretches thighs, knees, and ankles
- Strengthens core

Caution
- Knee issues
- Shoulder issues

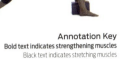

Annotation Key
Bold text indicates strengthening muscles
Black text indicates stretching muscles
* indicates deep muscles

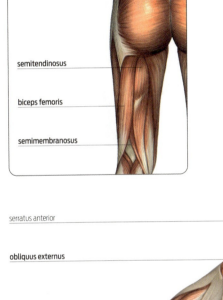

Back View

- gluteus medius*
- **semitendinosus**
- **biceps femoris**
- **semimembranosus**

triceps brachii

serratus anterior

obliquus externus

obliquus internus

vastus intermedius

vastus medialis

rectus femoris
vastus lateralis

35

ANATOMY OF FITNESS • YOGA

Half Moon Pose
(Ardha Chandrasana)

Half Moon Pose is a hip opener as well as a balancing posture. It also works as a strengthener for the entire core.

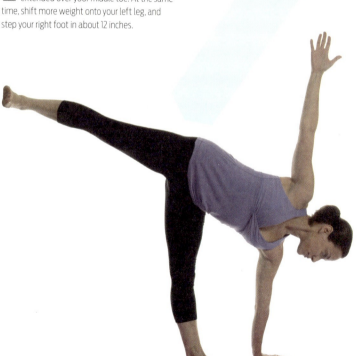

1 Stand in Extended Triangle Pose (pages 32–33) with your left palm or fingertips resting on your shin or on the floor. Gaze down toward your left foot, and bring your right hand onto your hip.

2 Bend your left knee slightly, keeping it extended over your middle toe. At the same time, shift more weight onto your left leg, and step your right foot in about 12 inches.

3 Straighten your left leg, opening the thigh while lifting your right leg to hip height. Keep your right leg in a neutral position, and flex your ankle.

4 Once you have your balance, extend your right arm straight up toward the ceiling, opening up across the front of your chest. Hold for 1 to 5 breaths. Repeat on the other side.

Half Moon Pose • **STANDING POSES**

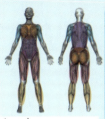

Correct form
- Gaze toward the floor, to the side, or up toward your raised hand.
- Imagine pressing your flexed foot into a wall behind you.

Avoid
- Letting your standing foot turn in.
- Allowing the knee of your standing foot to twist out of alignment.

Modifications
Easier: Rest your hand on a block if it is challenging for you to straighten your standing leg. You can turn the block on its side, depending on how limber you feel during your yoga practice.

Level
- Intermediate

Duration
- 1–5 breaths

Benefits
- Improves balance
- Opens hips
- Strengthens thighs, calves, and ankles

Caution
- Headache
- Low blood pressure

Annotation Key
Bold text indicates strengthening muscles
Black text indicates stretching muscles
* indicates deep muscles

- iliopsoas*
- transversus abdominis
- obliquus externus

- tensor fasciae latae
- latissimus dorsi
- serratus anterior
- rectus abdominis
- obliquus internus
- vastus medialis

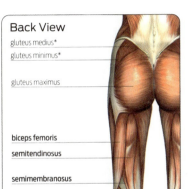

Back View
- gluteus medius*
- gluteus minimus*
- gluteus maximus
- biceps femoris
- semitendinosus
- semimembranosus

37

ANATOMY OF FITNESS • YOGA

Warrior I

(Virabhadrasana I)

Warrior I requires a mix of fortitude and flexibility. With practice, you will build strength and increase your confidence both on and off the mat.

1 Stand in the middle of your mat in Mountain Pose (pages 26–27), with your hands on your hips. Step or jump your feet about 3 to 4 feet apart. Turn your left toes out about 45 degrees so they face the upper left corner of your mat and walk your right foot to the right several inches until your feet are in heel-to-heel alignment.

2 Keeping your left leg straight, bend your right knee as you inhale, lifting your torso and arms above your head so that your upper body and arms form a straight line. Externally rotate both arms, palms facing each other, and energy up through your fingertips.

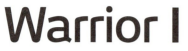

Correct form
- Reach up through your arms as you ground your feet down.
- Find a slight bend in your upper back.
- Keep your shoulders directly above your hips.

Avoid
- Twisting the knee of your back leg.

3 Hold the pose for 1 to 5 breaths with your shoulders, torso, and hips squared to the front of the mat. Your bent knee should stay in line with your middle toe, and your front thigh parallel to the floor. Press into the outer edge of your left foot and firm your left thigh as you slightly internally rotate the leg. Repeat on the other side.

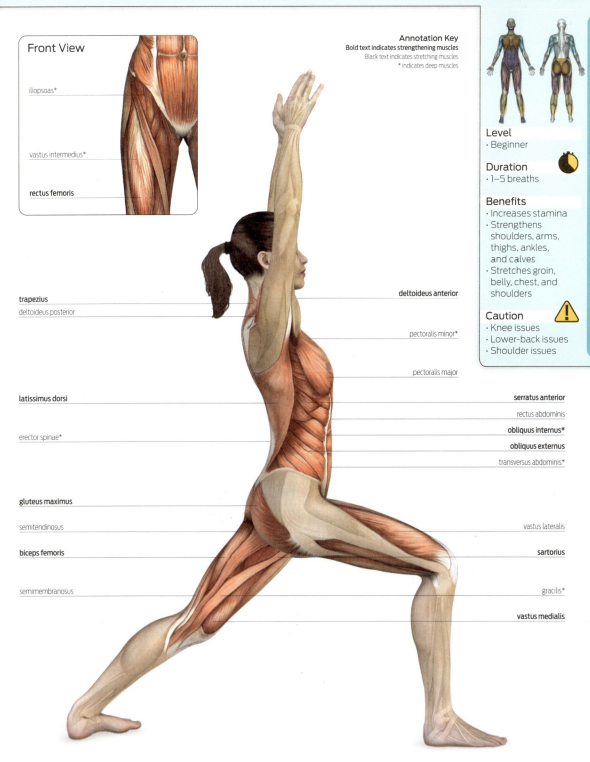

ANATOMY OF FITNESS • YOGA

Revolved Triangle Pose
(Parivrtta Trikonasana)

Revolved Triangle Pose can be very challenging because it requires hamstring and spine flexibility as well as stability and strength of the legs and hips.

1 Stand in the middle of your mat in Mountain Pose (pages 26–27). Place your hands on your hips, and step or jump your feet about 3 feet apart.

2 Turn your right toes about 45 degrees so they face the upper right corner of your mat, and walk your left foot to the left several inches, coming into heel-to-heel alignment.

3 Inhale both arms over your head into Upward Salute (pages 28–29). Exhale and bring your left hand to your left hip.

Correct form
- Keep your arms and legs straight.
- Use the inhalation to lengthen your spine, and the exhalation to twist.
- If you have tight hamstrings, widen your feet by walking your front foot closer to the edge of the mat, making sure your feet are not lined up as if you were on a tightrope.

Avoid
- Rounding your spine.

4 Inhale and extend your right arm as high as possible, finding length along the right side of your body, and hinge forward with a flat back as you twist to the left.

5 Place your right hand onto the floor on the outside of your left foot. Reach your left arm up to the ceiling, broadening across your collarbones.

6 Exhaling, twist the right side of your torso to the left and gaze toward the thumb of your upper hand.

7 Hold for 1 to 5 breaths. Continue to square your pelvis, and with each breath twist slightly deeper into the pose. Repeat on the other side.

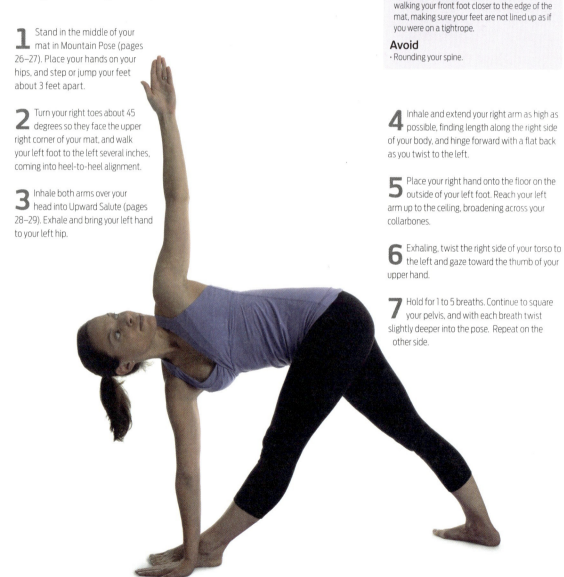

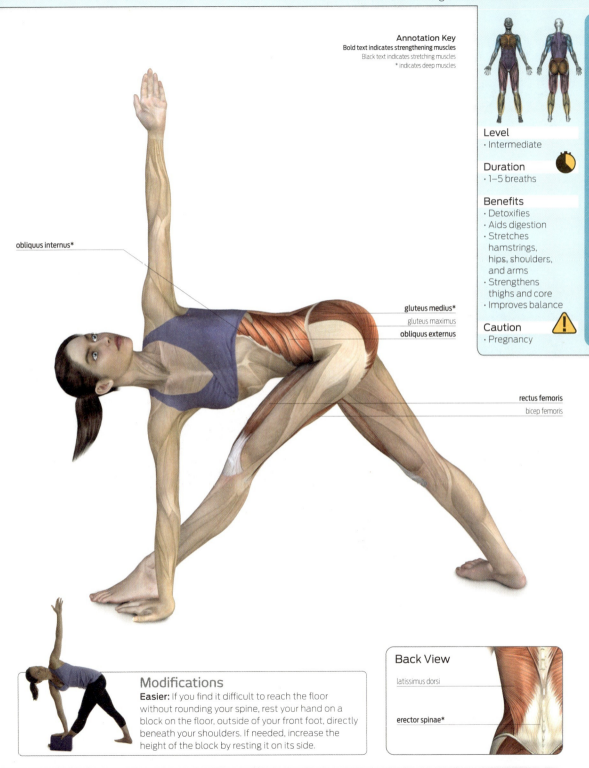

ANATOMY OF FITNESS • YOGA

Revolved Extended Side Angle Pose

(Parivrtta Parsvakonasana)

The full version of this pose can be quite challenging. If you find Revolved Extended Side Angle Pose too difficult at first, begin instead with an easier modification.

1 Stand in Mountain Pose (pages 26–27). Bring your hands to your hips, and with an exhale step or lightly jump your feet 3 to 4 feet apart.

2 Turn your left toes 45 degrees inward. Walk your right foot several inches to the right. Line your feet up so that they are in a heel-to-heel alignment.

3 Bring your hands together in a prayer position in front of your heart. Bend your right knee to that the thigh is parallel to the floor. Firm your left thigh, keeping the leg straight.

4 Twist your torso to the right, positioning your left elbow on the outside of your right thigh. Keep your hips square, drawing your right hip crease back.

5 Turn your gaze upward, and to the back right-hand corner of the room. Hold for 1 to 5 breaths, using the inhalation to lengthen your spine and the exhalation to twist more deeply. Repeat on the other side.

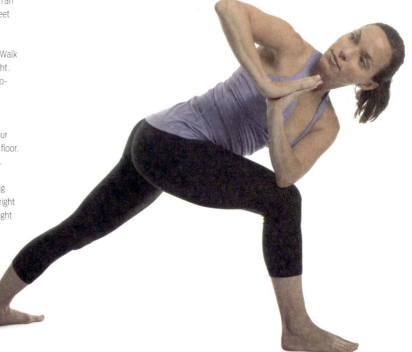

Modifications

Easier: Instead of keeping your back leg extended, bend it and rest your back knee and lower leg on the floor, making it easier to balance.

Easier: Instead of grounding your back foot into the floor, lift the heel. This will help you keep your hips squared.

Revolved Extended Side Angle Pose • **STANDING POSES**

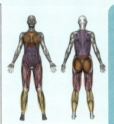

Correct form
- Keep your hands and arms in the prayer position as you twist.
- Your front foot should form a 90-degree angle with the front of your mat.
- Keep your front knee facing forward, in line with your middle toes.
- Press the pinky toe edge of your back foot firmly downward, and use the grounding of the back leg to help you twist.
- Resist your elbow into your thigh, and vice versa, to deepen the twist as you hold.

Avoid
- Letting your hips do the twisting; instead, keep them stable and squared to the front of your mat so that you can really twist from your spine.

Annotation Key
Bold text indicates strengthening muscles
Black text indicates stretching muscles
* indicates deep muscles

Level
- Intermediate/Advanced

Duration
- 1–5 breaths

Benefits
- Stretches hip, groin, torso, arms, and spine
- Strengthens thighs and ankles
- Detoxifies, helping with digestion and elimination
- Improves balance

Caution
- Pregnancy

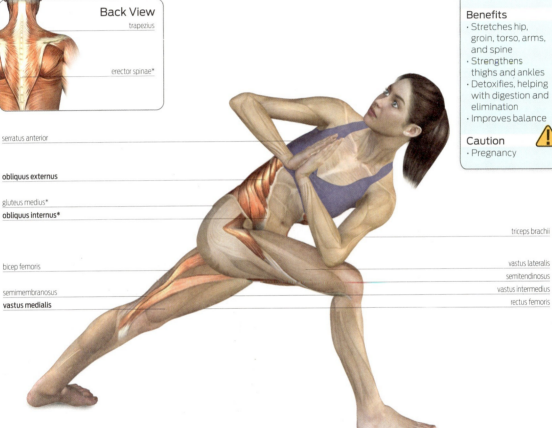

Back View
trapezius
erector spinae*

serratus anterior
obliquus externus
gluteus medius*
obliquus internus*
bicep femoris
semimembranosus
vastus medialis

triceps brachii
vastus lateralis
semitendinosus
vastus intermedius
rectus femoris

Modifications
Harder: Join your hands beneath your front leg.

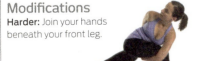

Same level of difficulty: Instead of keeping your hands and arms in the prayer position, place the hand of the arm opposite your front leg on the floor, and extend the other arm in line with your body, feeling a stretch along the side of your body.

ANATOMY OF FITNESS • YOGA

Warrior III
(Virabhadrasana III)

There are several different ways to come into Warrior III. You can start in Mountain Pose and step forward into the balancing position as an alternative to transitioning from Warrior I and High Lunge as described here.

1 Stand in Mountain Pose (pages 26–27). Step your right foot about 12 inches forward.

2 Extend your arms over your head, parallel to each other. Lift your left heel upward, shifting your weight onto the ball of your right foot.

3 Keep your left leg straight, pressing your left thigh up into the left hamstring to help energize it in preparation for lifting. Square your hips to the front of the mat, drawing your right hip back and your left hip forward. Keeping your arms extended over your head, hinge your torso forward over your right thigh.

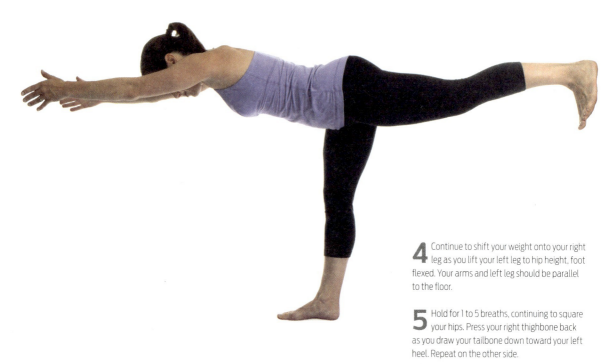

4 Continue to shift your weight onto your right leg as you lift your left leg to hip height, foot flexed. Your arms and left leg should be parallel to the floor.

5 Hold for 1 to 5 breaths, continuing to square your hips. Press your right thighbone back as you draw your tailbone down toward your left heel. Repeat on the other side.

Warrior III • **STANDING POSES**

Correct form
- Keep your hips squared.
- Keep length in the spine as you extend from your fingertips to your lifted heel.
- Energize your lifted leg to help you find balance.
- Ground down with the heel of your standing foot.

Avoid
- Allowing your lifted leg to bend or hang without control.

Annotation Key
Bold text indicates strengthening muscles
Black text indicates stretching muscles
* indicates deep muscles

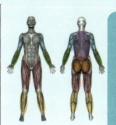

Level
- Intermediate/Advanced

Duration
- 1–5 breaths

Benefits
- Improves balance
- Strengthens ankles, calves, thighs, spine, core muscles, and shoulders
- Stretches thighs

Caution
- Lower-back issues

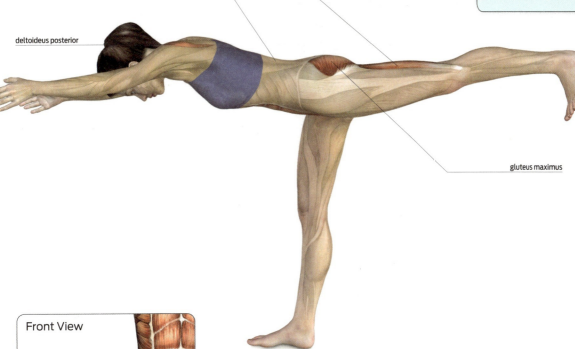

bicep femoris

erector spinae*

deltoideus posterior

gluteus maximus

Front View

rectus abdominis
obliquus internus*
transversus abdominis*

45

Revolved Half Moon Pose

(Parivrtta Ardha Chandrasana)

The counterpose to Half Moon Pose, Revolved Half Moon is a balancing pose as well as a twist. Holding this pose demands a great deal of core strength.

1 Begin in Revolved Triangle Pose (pages 40–41) with your legs about 3½ feet apart, your left hand on the floor on the outside of the right foot and your right arm reaching straight up.

2 Bring your right hand onto your right hip. Staying in the twist, turn your gaze toward the floor and bend your right knee slightly as you step your left foot about 12 inches in toward your right, shortening the stance. Lift your left leg up to hip height as you straighten your right standing leg.

3 Keep your hips squared to the floor as you twist your left ribs to the right. Once you have your balance, extend your right arm up to the ceiling. Externally rotate your arm and reach up through the fingertips.

4 Hold for 1 to 5 breaths. Continue to square your hips, drawing your right hip crease back and your left down toward the floor. Repeat on the other side.

Correct form
- Energize your lifted leg to help you balance; imagine that you are pressing your lifted foot against a wall.
- While holding, find a comfortable gazing point either at the floor or to the side before eventually turning your gaze up to your thumb.

Avoid
- Allowing the hip on the side of your lifted leg to drop toward the floor.

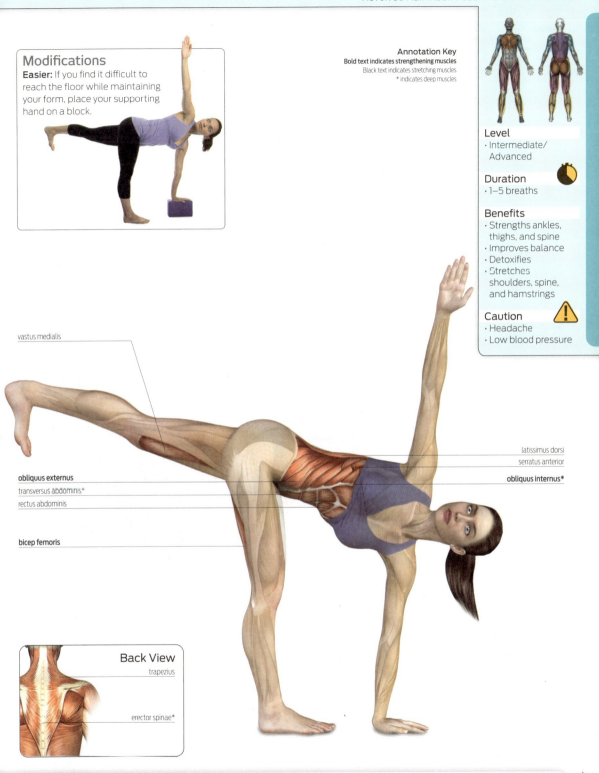

ANATOMY OF FITNESS • YOGA

Garland Pose
(Malasana)

Garland Pose is a great hip and inner thigh opener. If you are pregnant, this is a beneficial pose that you can practice throughout your entire pregnancy.

1 Stand in Mountain Pose (pages 26–27) facing the front short edge of your mat. Separate your feet wider than hip-distance apart.

2 Bend your knees as deeply as you can, letting your feet turn out, squatting down until your hips are lower than your knees.

3 Join your hands in a prayer position in front of your heart. Hold for 1 to 10 breaths.

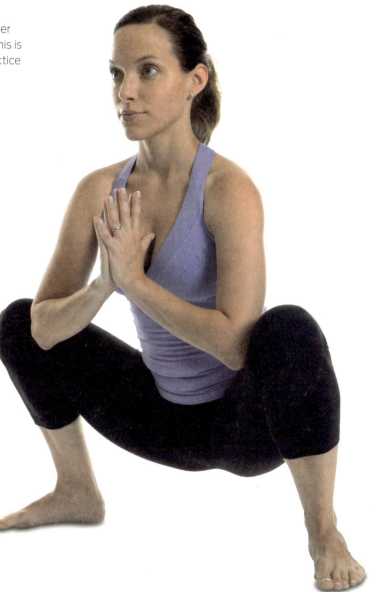

Correct form
- Use your elbows to apply gentle pressure on your knees, encouraging them to open further and deepening the inner thigh stretch.
- Resist your knees toward your elbows.
- If desired, place a blanket under your heels.
- Broaden across your collarbones.

Avoid
- Rounding your shoulders forward.

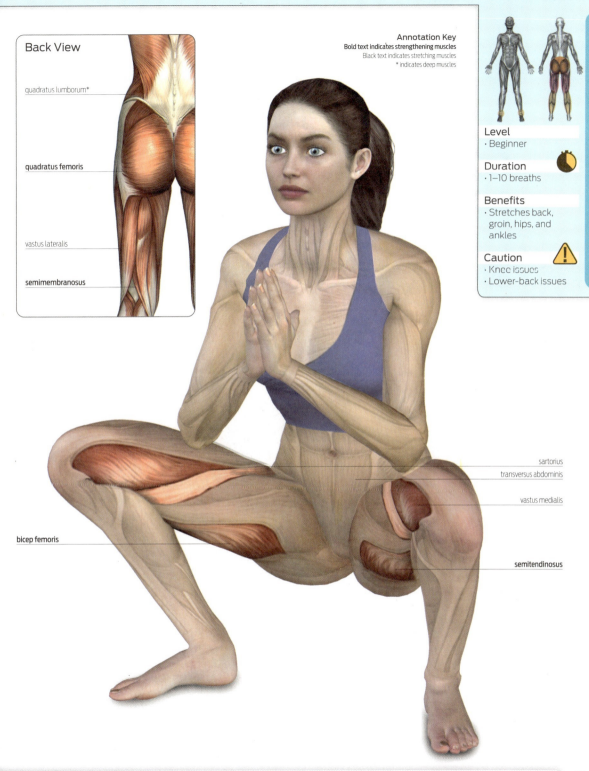

ANATOMY OF FITNESS • YOGA

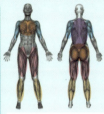

Level
• Beginner

Duration
• 1–5 breaths

Benefits
• Strengthens thighs, ankles, spine, and arms
• Stretches shoulders and chest

Caution
• Knee issues

Chair Pose
(Utkatasana)

You can easily control the intensity of Chair Pose, varying it by bending your knees just a few inches or all the way down so that your hips are in line with your knees. This pose is part of Sun Salutation B.

1 Begin in Mountain Pose (pages 26–27), with your feet together and arms by your sides. Inhale your arms into Upward Salute, reaching above your head so that your arms are parallel to each other. Rotate your outer upper arms inward and reach up through your fingertips.

Annotation Key
Black text indicates strengthening muscles
Gray text indicates stretching muscles
* indicates deep muscles

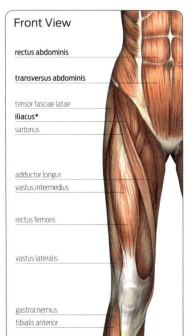

Front View
- rectus abdominis
- transversus abdominis
- tensor fasciae latae
- iliacus*
- sartorius
- adductor longus
- vastus intermedius
- rectus femoris
- vastus lateralis
- gastrocnemius
- tibialis anterior

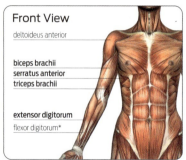

Front View
- deltoideus anterior
- biceps brachii
- serratus anterior
- triceps brachii
- extensor digitorum
- flexor digitorum*

2 Exhale, and bend your knees. Both ankles, inner thighs, and knees should be touching. Bring your weight onto your heels, try to shift your hips back, and draw your knees right above your ankles. Hold for 1 to 5 breaths.

Correct form
• Find a neutral position by drawing your tailbone down as you roll your inner thighs toward the floor.

Avoid
• Over-tucking your pelvis.
• Over-arching your lower back.
• Letting your feet separate or your knees knock inward.
• Lifting your heels.

Chair Pose and Twisting Chair Pose • **STANDING POSES**

Twisting Chair Pose
(Parivrtta Utkatasana)

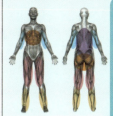

Twisting Chair Pose is great for improving digestion and elimination. Imagine wringing out your stomach as if it were a sponge, twisting a little deeper with each breath.

1 Begin in Chair Pose (page 50) with your arms parallel to each other above your head and your knees bent deeply.

2 Inhale as you lengthen your spine and join your hands in a prayer position in front of your heart.

3 Keep your hips square as you exhale and twist to the right, bringing your left elbow to the outside of your right thigh. Resist your left elbow into your right knee, and your knee into your elbow.

4 Inhale to lengthen the spine, letting your belly move outward, and then exhale to twist as your navel draws strongly back toward your spine. Hold for 1 to 5 breaths.

5 Inhaling, come to the center and reach your arms upward. Exhale as you begin to twist toward the left side, bringing your right elbow to the outside of your left thigh to repeat.

Level
· Intermediate

Duration
· 1–5 breaths

Benefits
· Detoxifies
· Strengthens thighs, ankles, spine, and arms
· Stretches spine
· Tones abdomen
· Helps with digestion

Caution
· Knee issues
· Pregnancy

Correct form
· Keep your hands in prayer position at the center of your chest, even though they will want to move toward one of your shoulders.
· Try to find a small bend in your upper back as you broaden across your collarbones.
· Twist from your torso and keep your hips square; if you are doing this, your knees will be in line with each other.

Avoid
· Rounding your shoulders as you twist.
· Twisting from your hips.
· Letting your left knee jut forward as you twist to the right, or vice versa.

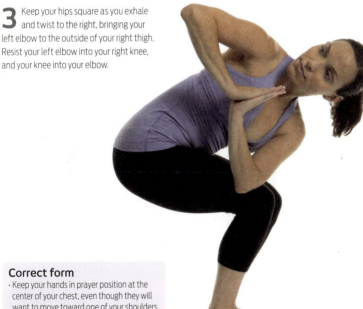

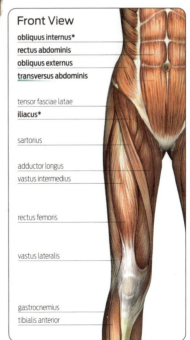

Front View

obliquus internus*
rectus abdominis
obliquus externus
transversus abdominis

tensor fasciae latae
iliacus*

sartorius

adductor longus
vastus intermedius

rectus femoris

vastus lateralis

gastrocnemius
tibialis anterior

Annotation Key
Bold text indicates strengthening muscles
Black text indicates stretching muscles
* indicates deep muscles

ANATOMY OF FITNESS • YOGA

Low Lunge
(Anjaneyasana)

Low Lunge can help to counteract soreness in the lower body. To come into the pose you can either step your foot forward from Downward-Facing Dog, as described here, or step your leg back from Standing Half Forward Bend.

1 Begin in Downward Facing Dog (pages 116–117). Exhale and step your right foot forward, planting it between your hands.

2 Drop your left knee and lower leg onto the floor, your toes extended along the floor behind you. You may need to walk the left knee back a few inches to deepen the stretch in the front of your left thigh and groin. Draw your tailbone down as your lift your frontal hipbones upward, finding a neutral pelvis.

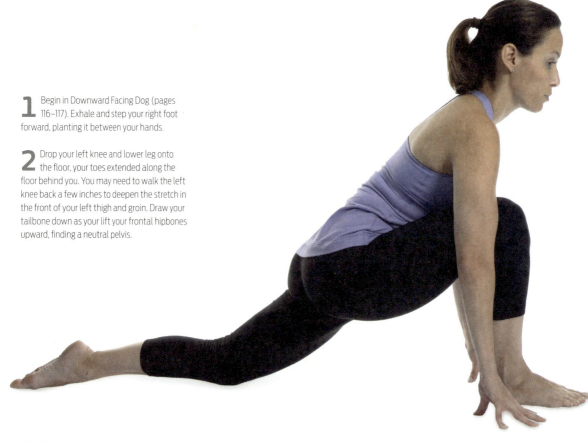

3 Slightly tuck your chin toward your chest to keep the back of the neck elongated. Hold for 1 to 5 breaths. Repeat on the other side.

Low Lunge • **STANDING POSES**

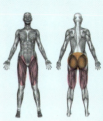

Front View

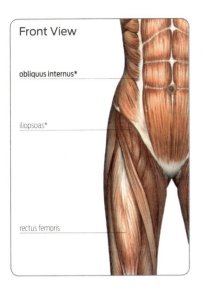

- obliquus internus*
- iliopsoas*
- rectus femoris

Correct form
- Position your front knee and shin directly above the ankle, with the center of your knee aligned with your middle toes.
- Shift your pelvis forward to deepen the stretch.
- Place a blanket under your knees if they feel sensitive.

Avoid
- Sinking into your lower back.
- Letting your front ribs pop forward.

Annotation Key
Bold text indicates strengthening muscles
Black text indicates stretching muscles
* indicates deep muscles

Level
- Beginner

Duration
- 1–5 breaths

Benefits
- Stretches thighs, hips, shoulders, chest, arms, and abdomen
- Strengthens thighs
- Tones hip abductor stabilizers

Caution
- Knee issues
- Lower-back issues

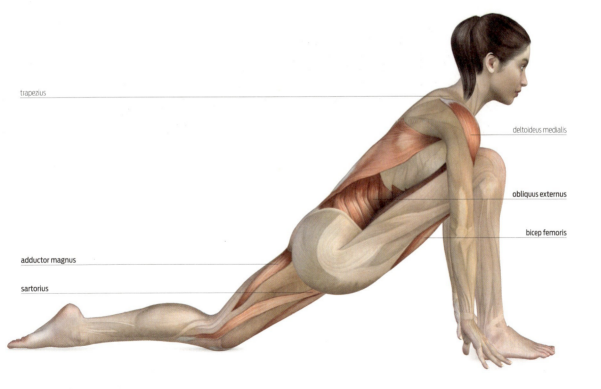

- trapezius
- adductor magnus
- sartorius
- deltoideus medialis
- obliquus externus
- bicep femoris

ANATOMY OF FITNESS • YOGA

High Lunge
(Prasarita Padottanasana)

High Lunge forms part of many yoga sequences, where it is often used as a way to step back to Downward-Facing Dog or as a way to step forward into Standing Forward Bend. Practiced on its own, it is an effective thigh strengthener.

1 From Downward-Facing Dog (pages 116–117), step your left foot forward in between your hands, with your left knee and shin lined up over your left ankle.

2 With your fingertips resting on the floor, square your hips to the front of the mat, grounding your left heel into the floor and drawing your left hip crease back.

3 Extend your right leg straight behind you, resting the ball of your foot on the mat. Lengthen all the way from the crown of your head to your right heel. Gaze slightly ahead, keeping the back of your neck long. Hold for 1 to 5 breaths. Repeat on the other side.

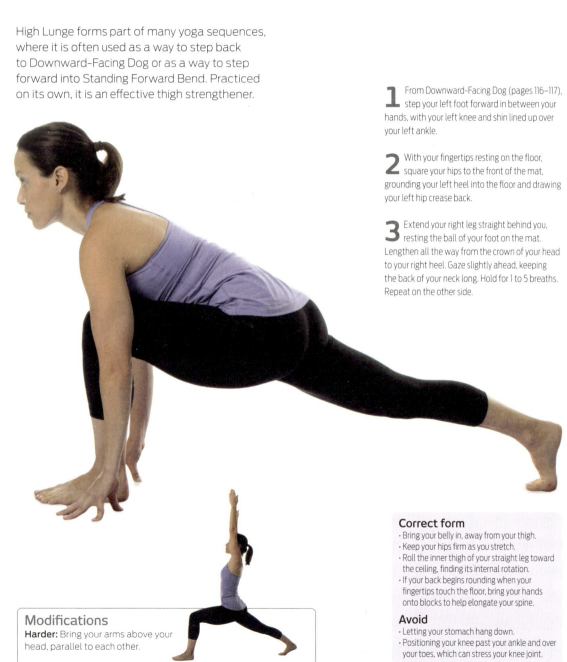

Modifications
Harder: Bring your arms above your head, parallel to each other.

Correct form
- Bring your belly in, away from your thigh.
- Keep your hips firm as you stretch.
- Roll the inner thigh of your straight leg toward the ceiling, finding its internal rotation.
- If your back begins rounding when your fingertips touch the floor, bring your hands onto blocks to help elongate your spine.

Avoid
- Letting your stomach hang down.
- Positioning your knee past your ankle and over your toes, which can stress your knee joint.

High Lunge • **STANDING POSES**

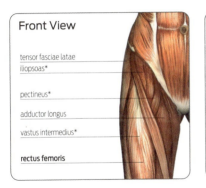
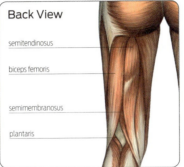
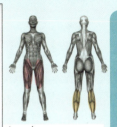

Level
· Beginner

Duration
· 1–5 breaths

Benefits
· Strengthens thighs
· Stretches hip flexors, shoulders, and chest
· With arms lifted, improves balance

Caution
· Knee issues

Annotation Key
Bold text indicates strengthening muscles
Black text indicates stretching muscles
* indicates deep muscles

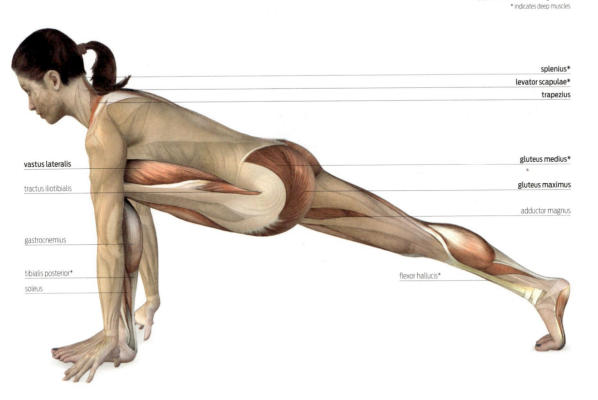

55

ANATOMY OF FITNESS • YOGA

Standing Split Pose

(Urdhva Prasarita Eka Padasana)

Unless you've had serious dance training, you've probably never done a standing split! Do not be intimidated—the purpose of this pose is to stretch the legs, not to achieve a 180-degree angle.

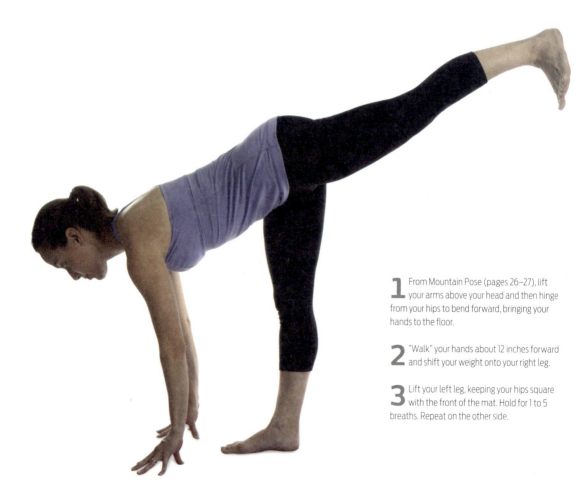

1 From Mountain Pose (pages 26–27), lift your arms above your head and then hinge from your hips to bend forward, bringing your hands to the floor.

2 "Walk" your hands about 12 inches forward and shift your weight onto your right leg.

3 Lift your left leg, keeping your hips square with the front of the mat. Hold for 1 to 5 breaths. Repeat on the other side.

Standing Split Pose • **STANDING POSES**

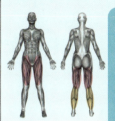

Annotation Key
Bold text indicates strengthening muscles
Black text indicates stretching muscles
* indicates deep muscles

Level
• Intermediate

Duration
• 1–5 breaths

Benefits
• Stretches thighs, groin, and hamstrings
• Strengthens thighs, calves, ankles, and knees
• Improves balance

Caution
• Ankle issues
• Knee issues
• Lower-back issues

Modifications
Harder: Try balancing while grasping the ankle of your standing foot with your hands. Allow the hip of your lifted leg to externally rotate.

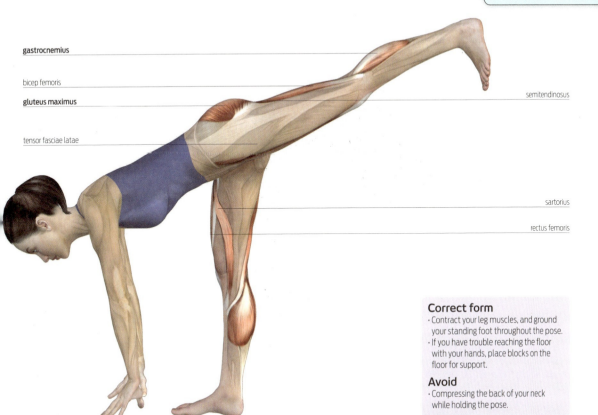

gastrocnemius

bicep femoris

gluteus maximus

tensor fasciae latae

semitendinosus

sartorius

rectus femoris

Correct form
• Contract your leg muscles, and ground your standing foot throughout the pose.
• If you have trouble reaching the floor with your hands, place blocks on the floor for support.

Avoid
• Compressing the back of your neck while holding the pose.

57

ANATOMY OF FITNESS • YOGA

Tree Pose
(Vrksasana)

In Tree Pose, as your standing foot stays strongly rooted to the floor, and the top of your head reaches up toward the ceiling, you will feel energy moving down and up at the same time.

1 From Mountain Pose (pages 26–27), bend your right knee, and bring your foot up to your left inner thigh, with toes pointing to the floor.

2 Externally rotate your right thigh, allowing your right knee to point out to the right while keeping your hips level.

3 Continue to open your right hip, rotating your inner thigh clockwise as you draw your tailbone down toward your left heel to neutralize your pelvis. Press your right foot into your left inner thigh as you draw your left outer hip in for stability.

4 Find your balance, and then join your hands in a prayer position. Hold for 1 to 5 breaths. Repeat on the other leg.

Modifications
Harder: Bring your hands above your head as you balance.

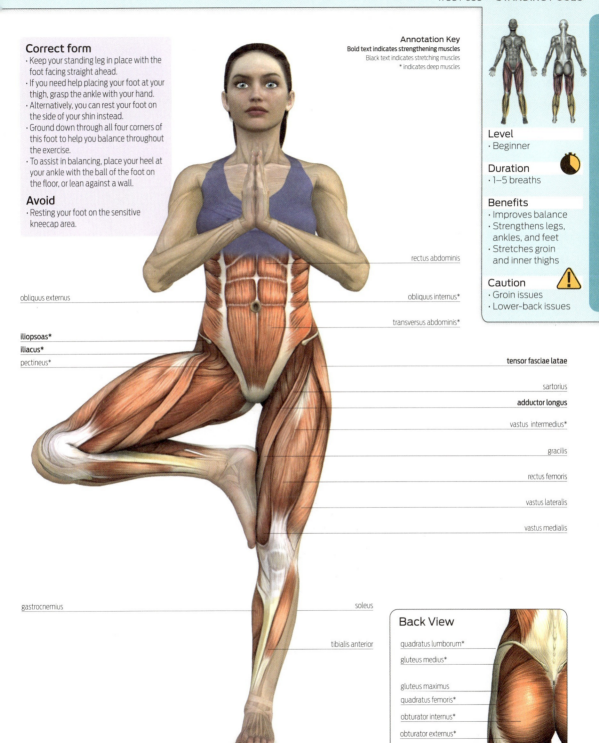

ANATOMY OF FITNESS • YOGA

Eagle Pose
(Garudasana)

Eagle Pose builds stamina and endurance. It is also an excellent pose for lubricating your joints.

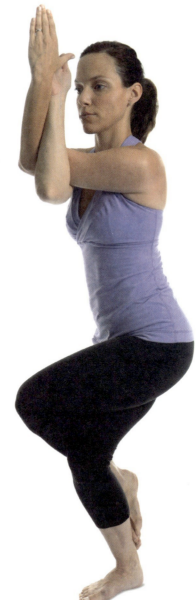

1 Stand in Mountain Pose (pages 26–27), and then bend your knees and sit into Chair Pose (page 50). Extend your arms out to your sides.

2 Keep your right knee bent in the chair position as you shift your weight onto your right heel. Lift your left knee into your chest and wrap the left thigh over your right thigh. If possible, wrap your left toes around the calf of your right leg.

3 Bring your arms in front of you with the palms facing up, bend your elbows, and hook your right elbow underneath your left elbow. Wrap your right forearm around your left and bring your palms together with your fingers pointing toward the ceiling.

4 Squeeze your arms together and lift your elbows up as you bring your hands away from your face to broaden across your upper back. Hold for 1 to 5 breaths. Repeat on the other side.

Correct form
- Squeeze your inner thighs together as you draw your tailbone down toward the floor and lift your frontal hip bones up.
- If you have trouble balancing, bring your raised foot to the floor on the outside of the standing foot.
- Find a fixed gazing point, keeping your eyes soft.

Avoid
- Letting your hips twist to either side.

Eagle Pose • **STANDING POSES**

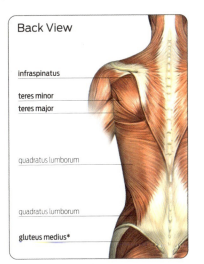

Back View

- infraspinatus
- teres minor
- teres major
- quadratus lumborum
- quadratus lumborum
- gluteus medius*

Annotation Key
Bold text indicates strengthening muscles
Black text indicates stretching muscles
* indicates deep muscles

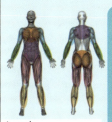

Level
- Beginner/ Intermediate

Duration
- 1–5 breaths

Benefits
- Helps to release tension in upper back
- Stretches hips and buttocks
- Strengthens thighs, ankles, and knees
- Builds stamina and endurance
- Improves concentration

Caution
- Groin issues
- Knee issues

- serratus anterior
- rectus femoris
- adductor magnus

- trapezius
- coracobrachialis
- latissimus dorsi
- gluteus maximus

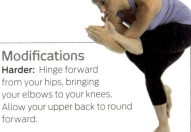

Modifications
Harder: Hinge forward from your hips, bringing your elbows to your knees. Allow your upper back to round forward.

61

ANATOMY OF FITNESS • YOGA

Extended Hand-to-Big-Toe Pose

(Utthita Hasta Padangusthasana)

When performing Extended Hand-to-Big-Toe Pose, focus on grounding your standing leg: keep it straight, with your spine long, and then extend your leg. Allow yourself enough time to find your balance; on some days, you will find yourself being better able to balance than on others.

1 Stand in Mountain Pose (pages 26–27). Shift some of your weight onto your left foot as you bend your right knee into your chest, placing your left hand on your hip.

2 Grab your right toe in yogic toe lock, with your index finger and middle finger wrapped around the inside of the big toe, and your thumb wrapped around the outside of the toe.

3 Slightly internally rotate your left thigh and firm the whole leg. Exhaling, extend your right leg forward, aiming to straighten it. Hold for 1 to 5 breaths. Repeat on the other side.

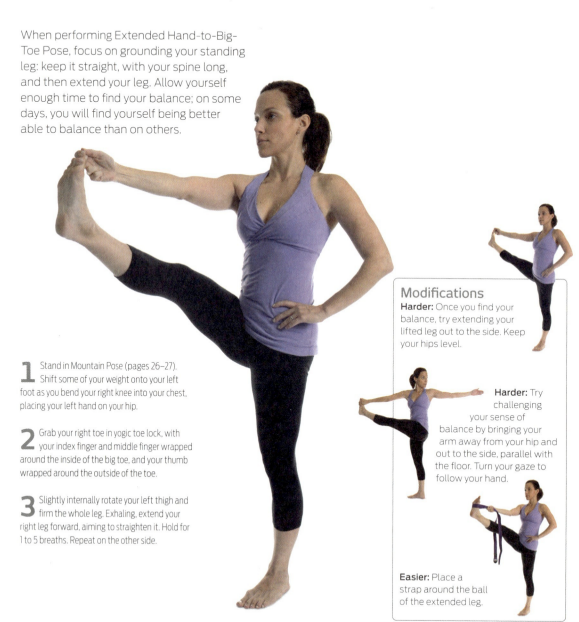

Modifications

Harder: Once you find your balance, try extending your lifted leg out to the side. Keep your hips level.

Harder: Try challenging your sense of balance by bringing your arm away from your hip and out to the side, parallel with the floor. Turn your gaze to follow your hand.

Easier: Place a strap around the ball of the extended leg.

Extended Hand-to-Big-Toe Pose • **STANDING POSES**

Correct form
- If you find yourself leaning your torso forward and rounding your back to straighten your leg, then keep it bent; it is more important to elongate your spine than to straighten your extended leg.
- On the side of your lifted leg, draw your hip crease back to keep your hips square.
- Keep your spine upright with your shoulders in line over your hips.
- Ground the heel of your standing leg into the floor to maintain your balance.
- Take your time in finding your balance.
- Keep your standing leg straight.

Avoid
- Letting your hip lift upward in an attempt to raise your leg.
- Locking the knee of your standing leg.
- Allowing your shoulder to protract forward as you hold your toe.
- Twisting your hips.

Annotation Key
Bold text indicates strengthening muscles
Black text indicates stretching muscles
* indicates deep muscles

Level
- Intermediate

Duration
- 1–5 breaths

Benefits
- Strengthens spine, legs, and ankles
- Stretches hamstrings and shoulders
- Improves balance

Caution
- Ankle issues
- Foot issues
- Lower-back issues

palmaris longus
flexor carpi radialis
pronator teres
semimembranosus
bicep femoris
semitendinosus
vastus medialis
gracilis*
vastus lateralis
rectus femoris
tibialis anterior

Back View
quadratus lumborum
piriformis
gemellus superior*
gluteus maximus
gemellus inferior*

ANATOMY OF FITNESS • YOGA

Lord of the Dance Pose

(Natarajasana)

Lord of the Dance Pose is a powerful balancing pose. Nataraja is another name for Shiva the Lord of the Dance, whose name is associated with creation and destruction of the world.

1 Begin in Mountain Pose (pages 26–27). Keeping your knees together, bend your left knee and draw your heel toward your buttocks. Grasp the inside of your foot with your left hand.

2 Reach your right arm up to the ceiling so that the upper arm is next to your ear. Begin to lift your left knee up behind you, keeping your hips square.

3 Bring your right arm slightly forward and raise your left leg even higher, pressing your foot and your hand together.

4 Find a gazing point either about 5 feet in front of you, on the floor, or on the horizon as you find your balance. Hold for 1 to 5 breaths. Repeat on the other side.

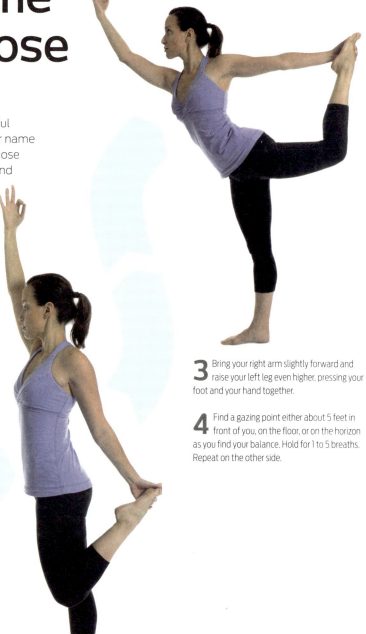

Lord of the Dance Pose • **STANDING POSES**

Annotation Key
Bold text indicates strengthening muscles
Black text indicates stretching muscles
* indicates deep muscles

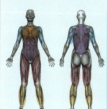

Level
- Intermediate

Duration
- 1–5 breaths

Benefits
- Stretches chest, abdomen, shoulders, thighs, hips, groin, and ankles
- Strengthens legs and ankles
- Improves balance

Caution
- Ankle issues
- Foot issues
- Lower-back issues

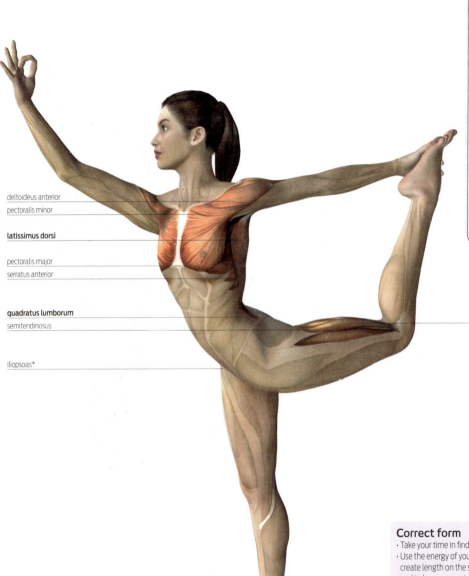

- deltoideus anterior
- pectoralis minor
- **latissimus dorsi**
- pectoralis major
- serratus anterior
- **quadratus lumborum**
- semitendinosus
- iliopsoas*
- bicep femoris

Correct form
- Take your time in finding your balance.
- Use the energy of your arm reaching up to create length on the same side of the body, and to keep your spine as upright as possible.
- Bend from your upper back.

Avoid
- Leaning your torso too far forward as you lift your leg.

ANATOMY OF FITNESS • YOGA

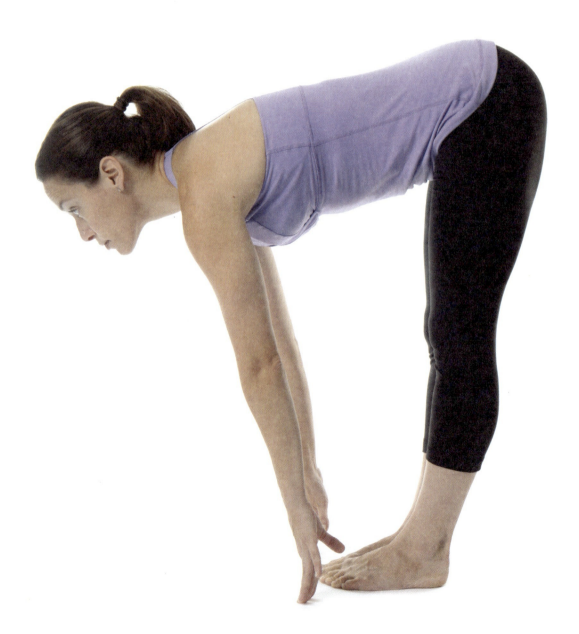

Standing Forward Bends

Standing Forward Bends have many benefits. Thought to calm the central nervous system, help to alleviate symptoms of mild depression, and heal headaches, these poses will really stretch your hamstrings, calves, ankles, hips, and lower back. Because these bends are weight-bearing, they also help to strengthen your legs and stabilize your hips. And as your head releases downward, tension in your upper back, shoulders, and neck dissipates as your spine is stretched. While seated forward bends are often practiced at the end of the yoga session, standing forward bends tend to be dispersed throughout the session.

Contents

Cat Pose	68
Intense Side Stretch	70
Standing Half Forward Bend to Standing Forward Bend	72
Wide-Legged Forward Bend	74

ANATOMY OF FITNESS • YOGA

Cat Pose
(Marjaryana)

Cat Pose and Cow Pose (pages 78–79) are often practiced together in a sequence that flows from one pose to the other, helping to connect the body with the breath. Inhale to extend your spine into Cow, and then exhale to round it into Cat.

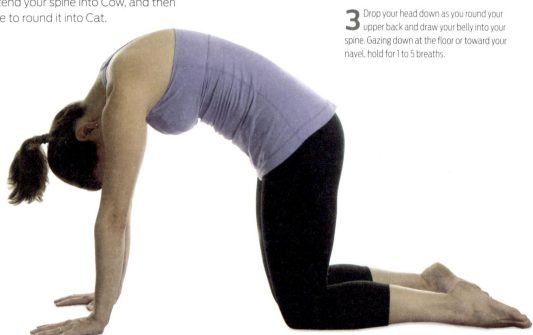

3 Drop your head down as you round your upper back and draw your belly into your spine. Gazing down at the floor or toward your navel, hold for 1 to 5 breaths.

1 Begin on your hands and knees with your hands shoulder distance apart and your knees hip distance apart, with the tops of your feet on the floor. Align your wrists directly beneath your shoulders and your knees below your hips. Find a neutral pelvis, neither tucking it nor arching your lower back.

2 Spread your fingers wide, grounding down through your thumb and index fingers. Externally rotate your arms, thinking of opening your right upper arm clockwise and your left upper arm counterclockwise.

Correct form
- Allow your shoulder blades to separate and breathe more space into your upper spine.
- Keep your shoulders over your wrists as you round your back.

Avoid
- Bringing the weight back toward your knees as you round your spine.

Cat Pose • STANDING FORWARD BENDS

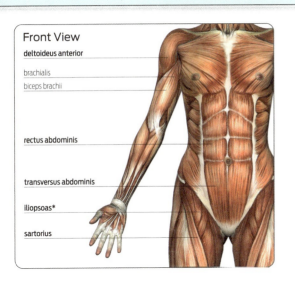

Front View
- deltoideus anterior
- brachialis
- biceps brachii
- rectus abdominis
- transversus abdominis
- iliopsoas*
- sartorius

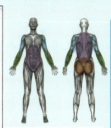

Level
- Beginner

Duration
- 1–5 breaths

Benefits
- Stretches neck and spine
- Strengthens abdomen and arms

Caution
- Knee issues

Annotation Key
Bold text indicates strengthening muscles
Black text indicates stretching muscles
* indicates deep muscles

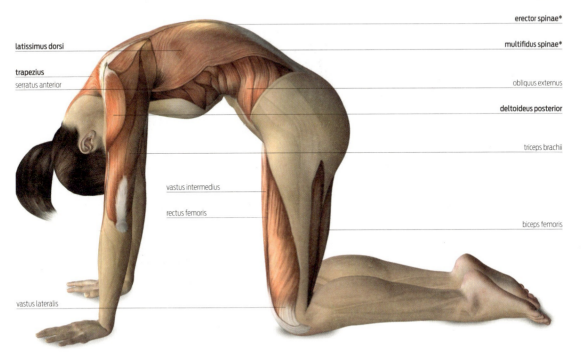

- latissimus dorsi
- **trapezius**
- serratus anterior
- vastus intermedius
- rectus femoris
- vastus lateralis
- erector spinae*
- multifidus spinae*
- obliquus externus
- **deltoideus posterior**
- triceps brachii
- biceps femoris

69

Intense Side Stretch

(Parsvottanasana)

Intense Side Stretch is a forward bend that is calming. It also provides an intense stretch for your hamstrings—especially beneficial if you like to run.

1 From Mountain Pose (pages 26–27), step your left foot back about 3 feet. Turn your toes in about 45 degrees so that they face the upper left corner of your mat. Come into heel-to-heel alignment, squaring your hips to the front of the mat.

2 Extend your arms out parallel to the floor, turn your thumbs down, bend your elbows, and join your hands into a prayer position: begin with the backs of your hands together and the fingers pointing down, and then turn your fingers away from your back and flip your wrists so that your fingers point upward. Press your pinky fingers together, and slowly try to press your hands together.

3 Inhale, broadening across your collarbones, drawing your shoulder blades together and lifting your chest while keeping your hips squared.

4 Ground through the pinky toe edge of your left foot, and press your left thigh back as you exhale to fold forward over your right leg. Lead with your heart and keep your spine elongated. Hold for 1 to 5 breaths.

5 Inhale, draw your shoulders back, and lift your sternum, leading with your heart to come up to standing. Step your left foot forward to meet your right foot in Mountain Pose, and repeat on the other side.

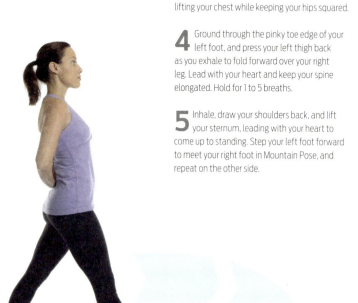
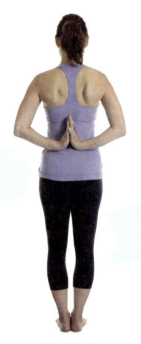

Intense Side Stretch • **STANDING FORWARD BENDS**

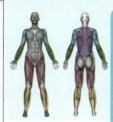

Front View

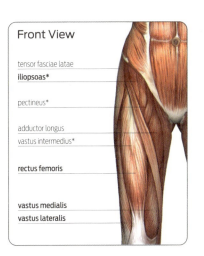

- tensor fasciae latae
- **iliopsoas***
- pectineus*
- adductor longus
- vastus intermedius*
- **rectus femoris**
- **vastus medialis**
- **vastus lateralis**

Correct form
- As you square your hips, draw your right hip crease back as you press your right big toe to counteract that movement. (Reverse these instructions when performing on the other side.)
- If you have tight hamstrings, try widening your stance by walking your front foot closer to the right edge of the mat.

Avoid
- Rounding your back as you fold forward.

Annotation Key
Bold text indicates strengthening muscles
Black text indicates stretching muscles
* indicates deep muscles

Level
- Beginner/ Intermediate

Duration
- 1–5 breaths

Benefits
- Strengthens legs and spine
- Stretches legs, spine, shoulders, and wrists
- Improves posture
- Calms mind and body

Caution
- Hamstring issues
- Spine issues

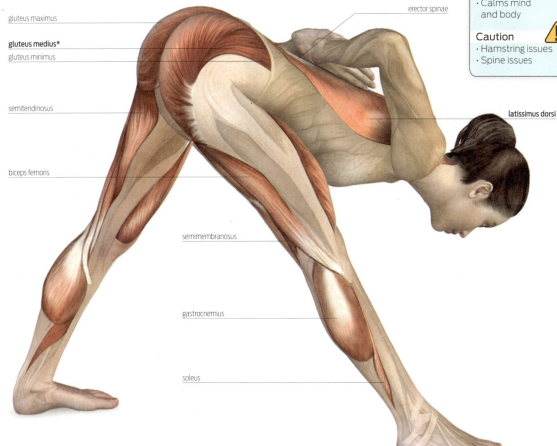

- gluteus maximus
- **gluteus medius***
- gluteus minimus
- semitendinosus
- biceps femoris
- erector spinae
- **latissimus dorsi**
- semimembranosus
- gastrocnemius
- soleus

Standing Half Forward Bend to Standing Forward Bend

(Ardha Uttanasana to Uttanasana)

Often repeated throughout yoga classes, Standing Half Forward Bend and Standing Forward Bend form part of the Sun Salutation sequences. Each time you perform these poses, you will fold a little deeper into the forward bend.

1 From Mountain Pose (pages 26–27), inhale and raise both arms toward the ceiling. Exhale as you hinge at the hips to fold forward, bringing your arms down until your fingertips reach the floor. Spread out your toes and press down evenly through all four corners of your feet. Plant your fingertips in line with your toes and look forward.

2 Straighten your legs and arms as you lift your chest up away from your legs. Broaden across the front of your chest, finding a slight backward bend in your upper back as you draw your stomach in.

3 Press your heels into the floor as you lift your tailbone up toward the ceiling, keeping your hips in line with your heels. This is Standing Half Forward Bend.

4 Inhale to lengthen your spine, then exhale as you fold forward from your hips and bring your fingertips or palms to the floor. This is Standing Forward Bend.

5 Lengthen your torso as you bring your belly closer to your thighs, ground your heels into the floor, and lift your tailbone toward the ceiling. Hold for 1 to 5 breaths, inhaling to lengthen your spine and exhaling to fold deeper.

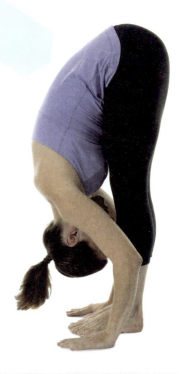

Standing Half Forward Bend to Standing Forward Bend • **STANDING FORWARD BENDS**

Correct form
- Keep a slight bend in your knees if you have a tight lower back or hamstrings. Separating your feet hip-width apart also helps if you have tight hamstrings.
- If you can't reach the floor during Standing Half Forward Bend, place your hands on your shins.
- If you cannot reach the floor during Standing Forward Bend, place your hands on blocks or bend your arms and hold opposite elbows.

Avoid
- Shifting your weight backward so that your hips are behind your heels.

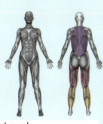

Level
- Beginner

Duration
- 1–5 breaths

Benefits
- Stretches hamstrings, hips, and spine
- Strengthens thighs and knees
- Reduces stress
- Aids digestion

Caution
- Lower-back issues

Annotation Key
Bold text indicates strengthening muscles
Black text indicates stretching muscles
* indicates deep muscles

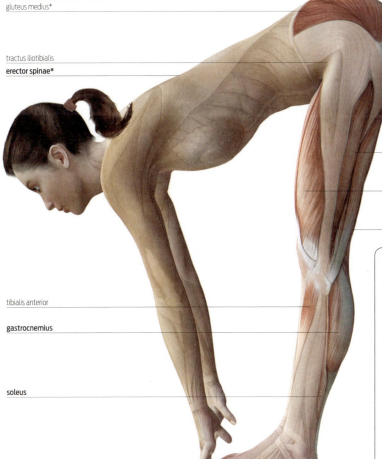

piriformis*
gluteus medius*
tractus iliotibialis
erector spinae*
tibialis anterior
gastrocnemius
soleus

gluteus maximus
semitendinosus
biceps femoris
vastus lateralis
semimembranosus

Front View

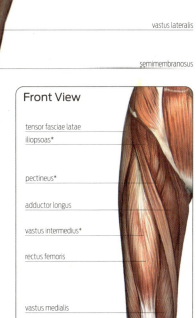

tensor fasciae latae
iliopsoas*
pectineus*
adductor longus
vastus intermedius*
rectus femoris
vastus medialis

73

Wide-Legged Forward Bend

(Prasarita Padottanasana)

Wide-Legged Forward Bend is a great stretch for your hamstrings and spine. It is also technically an inversion, as your head is positioned below your heart.

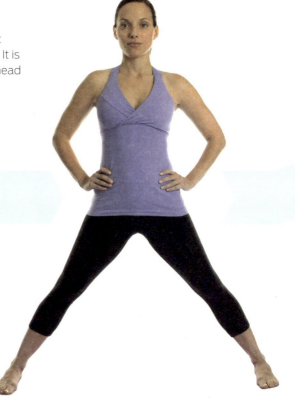

1 Stand in the middle of your mat in Mountain Pose (pages 26–27) with your hands on your hips. Step or jump your feet so that they are parallel, 3 to 4 feet apart.

2 On an inhalation, lengthen your spine, lift your chest, and find a slight bend in your upper back, bringing your gaze up to the ceiling.

3 Exhaling, hinge forward from your hips until your palms are on the floor, with your fingers facing forward. Walk your hands back until your hands are in line with your heels. Bring the crown of your head toward the floor, lifting your shoulders toward your ears to make space for your neck.

Correct form
- Keep your knees soft.
- Hinge forward with your chest open and your back flat.
- Bend only as far forward as you can go while maintaining your flat back.
- Keep your hips lined up above your heels. (To this end, it helps to shift your weight onto the balls of your feet.)

Avoid
- Rounding your back to place your hands on the floor.
- Locking your knees.

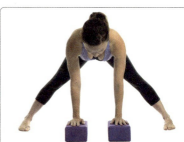

Modifications
Easier: If you find it difficult to reach the floor with your hands, place some blocks on the floor and reach for them instead.

Wide-Legged Forward Bend • STANDING FORWARD BENDS

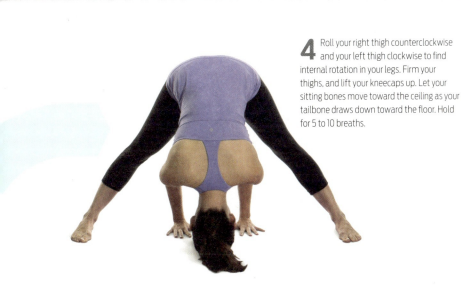

4 Roll your right thigh counterclockwise and your left thigh clockwise to find internal rotation in your legs. Firm your thighs, and lift your kneecaps up. Let your sitting bones move toward the ceiling as your tailbone draws down toward the floor. Hold for 5 to 10 breaths.

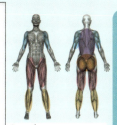

Level
• Beginner

Duration
• 5–10 breaths

Benefits
• Strengthens spine
• Stretches inner and outer hips
• Releases groin
• Calms mind and body

Caution
• Back issues
• Hamstring issues

Annotation Key
Bold text indicates strengthening muscles
Black text indicates stretching muscles
* indicates deep muscles

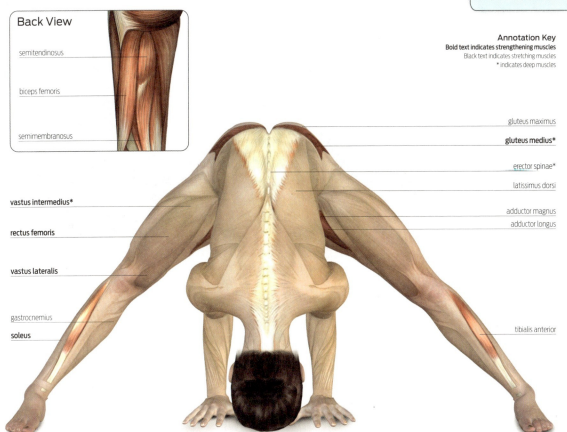

Back View
- semitendinosus
- biceps femoris
- semimembranosus

- **vastus intermedius***
- **rectus femoris**
- **vastus lateralis**
- gastrocnemius
- soleus

- gluteus maximus
- **gluteus medius***
- erector spinae*
- latissimus dorsi
- adductor magnus
- adductor longus
- tibialis anterior

ANATOMY OF FITNESS • YOGA

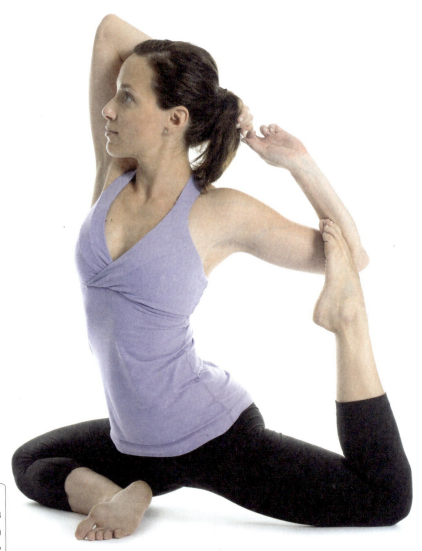

Contents

Cow Pose	78
Upward-Facing Dog	80
Cobra Pose	82
Locust Pose	84
Half-Frog Pose	86
Bow Pose	88
Bridge Pose	90
Wheel Pose	92
Camel Pose	94
Fish Pose	96
Pigeon Pose	98

Backbends

Backbends are often called heart openers. While the spine is bending backward, the entire front of the body—the chest, lungs, abdomen and internal organs—is being stretched open. Many people tend to hold tension in their upper back and neck, and/or to round their shoulders forward. Backbends help to release some of that built-up tension. They also improve posture by increasing the strength and flexibility of the spine. Backbends are invigorating; after practicing a backbend you will feel noticeably more energized.

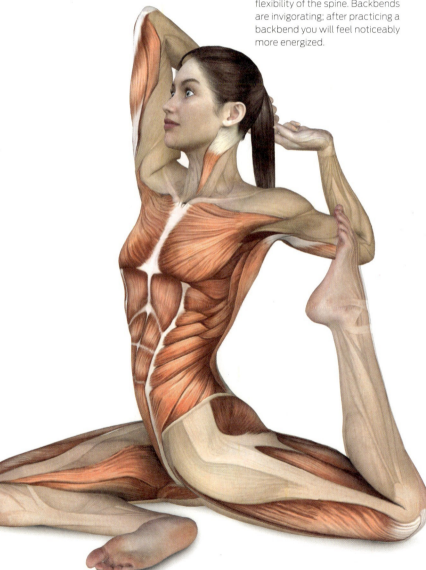

ANATOMY OF FITNESS • YOGA

Cow Pose

(Bitilasana)

Cow Pose is often accompanied by Cat Pose (pages 68–69). They are frequently linked together, with one breath per movement. Flowing gently between Cat and Cow is an easy way to warm up the spine.

1 Begin on your hands and knees, with your hands planted directly below your shoulders and your knees beneath your hips. Your hips should be in a neutral position.

2 Spread your fingers wide, grounding down through your knuckles.

3 On an inhalation, lift your sternum and arch your upper back, lifting your sitting bones toward the ceiling. Hold for 1 to 5 breaths.

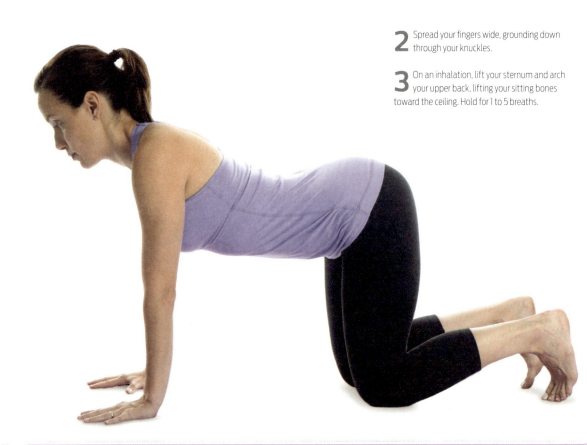

Cow Pose • **BACKBENDS**

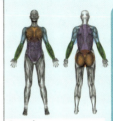

Correct form
- Arch your back and draw your stomach muscles toward your spine to keep from sinking in your lower back.

Avoid
- Letting your stomach hang down.

Annotation Key
Bold text indicates strengthening muscles
Black text indicates stretching muscles
* indicates deep muscles

Level
- Beginner

Duration
- 1–5 breaths

Benefits
- Stretches chest, neck, and spine

Caution
- Neck issues

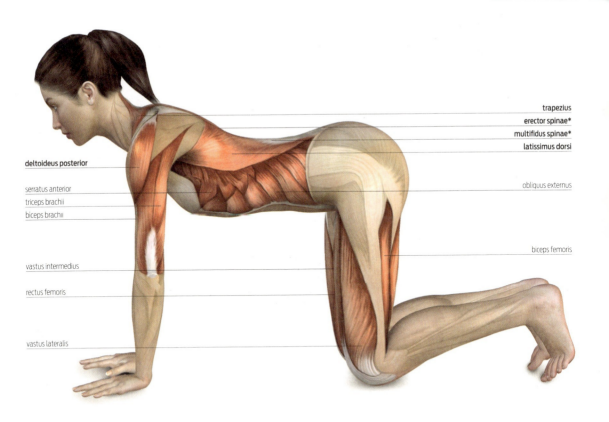

ANATOMY OF FITNESS • YOGA

Upward-Facing Dog
(Urdhva Mukha Svanasana)

Upward-Facing Dog helps to counteract the effects of hours spent hunched over computers and steering wheels. An effective backbend, it forms an important part of both Sun Salutations.

Correct form
- Keep your wrists parallel to the front edge of your mat.
- Position your shoulders above your wrists.
- Keep your chin tucked slightly as you lengthen the back of your neck.
- While holding the pose, focus on a comfortable gazing point, such as the spot where wall and ceiling meet.

Avoid
- Resting your thighs on the floor.
- Positioning your hands in front of your shoulders.
- Externally rotating your thighs, as this can compress your lower back.

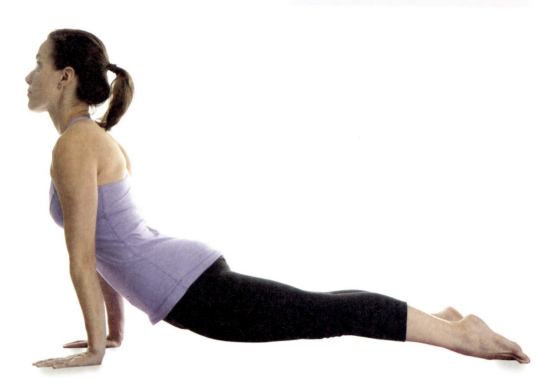

1 Lie facedown on your stomach. Bend your arms and place your wrists underneath your elbows, with your fingers facing toward the front of your mat.

2 Inhale and straighten your arms so that your shoulders are directly above your wrists as you lift your thighs and knees off the floor.

3 Spread your fingers, and ground down. Draw your tailbone down, and lift your pubic bone toward your belly button. Hold for 1 to 5 breaths.

Upward-Facing Dog • **BACKBENDS**

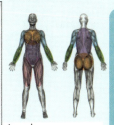

Front View
- serratus anterior
- rectus abdominis
- tensor fasciae latae
- iliopsoas*
- adductor longus
- vastus intermedius*
- rectus femoris
- vastus lateralis
- vastus medialis

Back View
- teres minor
- teres major
- rhomboideus*
- erector spinae*
- quadratus lumborum*
- gluteus medius*
- adductor magnus
- semitendinosus
- biceps femoris
- semimembranosus

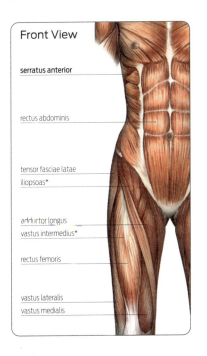
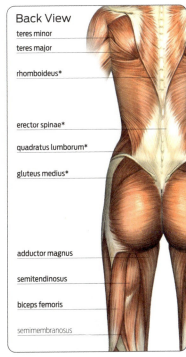

Level
- Beginner/Intermediate

Duration
- 1–5 breaths

Benefits
- Stretches shoulders, chest, abdomen, thighs, and ankles
- Strengthens wrists, arms, and spine
- Improves posture

Caution
- Lower-back issues
- Pregnancy
- Shoulder issues
- Wrist issues

Annotation Key
Bold text indicates strengthening muscles
Black text indicates stretching muscles
* indicates deep muscles

- sternocleidomastoideus
- latissimus dorsi
- triceps brachii
- gluteus maximus

81

Cobra Pose

(Bhujangasana)

Cobra Pose stretches and strengthens the spine. Don't try to lift your chest and shoulders too high at first; with this pose, there is power in small movement.

1 Lie facedown on your stomach. Bend your arms and place your wrists underneath your elbows, with your fingers facing toward the front of your mat. Draw your elbows in toward your body.

2 On an inhalation, press your hands into the floor and lift your chest and shoulders upward, drawing your sternum forward and your shoulder blades together.

3 Press into the floor with your toenails, especially those of your pinky toes, to help you find internal rotation in the thighs. Firm your buttocks. Straighten your legs and roll your inner thighs toward the ceiling. Feel your pubic bone pressing down to the floor as you draw your tailbone down toward your feet. Hold for 1 to 5 breaths.

4 Lead with your forehead as you lower yourself back to the mat on an exhalation.

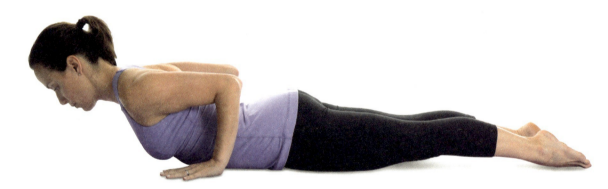

Correct form
- Keep the back of your neck long.
- Draw your belly button toward your spine even though your stomach is resting on the floor.

Avoid
- Turning your legs outward.
- Lifting your feet off the floor as your raise your chest.
- Squeeze your buttocks so hard that your lower back feels tense or crunched.

Cobra Pose • **BACKBENDS**

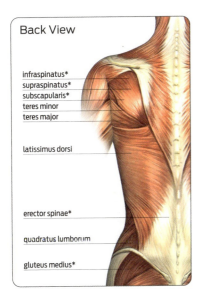

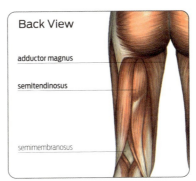

Annotation Key
Bold text indicates strengthening muscles
Black text indicates stretching muscles
* indicates deep muscles

Level
• Beginner

Duration
• 1–5 breaths

Benefits
• Stretches and strengthens spine and upper arms
• Stretches front of body
• Improves posture

Caution
• Lower-back issues
• Pregnancy

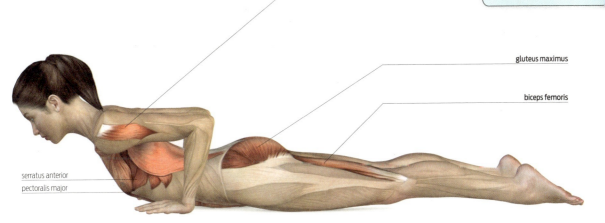

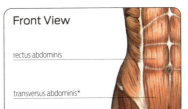

83

Locust Pose

(Salabhasana)

Locust Pose will strengthen the entire back of your body as well as your core muscles. It is great preparation for deeper backbends.

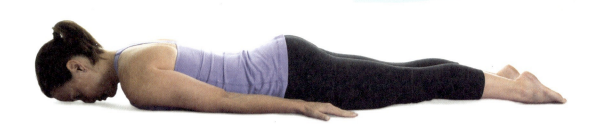

1 Lie on your stomach, with your arms and legs extended straight behind you and your forehead resting on the floor. Press every toenail into the floor, especially those of your pinky toes, to encourage internal rotation in your legs.

2 On an inhalation, lift your head, chest, legs, and arms up off the floor.

Correct form
- If desired, try interlacing your fingers behind your back or extending your arms forward.
- If your hip bones feel sensitive, place a blanket under your pelvis.
- Gaze slightly forward to maintain length in the back of your neck.

Avoid
- Twisting or crunching the back of your neck.

Locust Pose • **BACKBENDS**

3 Continue to internally rotate your thighs by rolling your inner thighs toward the ceiling as your tailbone draws down toward your feet and your hip bones lift toward your belly button. Lengthen all four sides of your torso to help lift your sternum and shoulders away from the floor. Hold for 3 to 5 breaths.

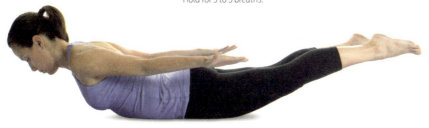

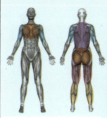

Level
• Beginner

Duration
• 3–5 breaths

Benefits
• Tones and strengthens spine, buttocks, hamstrings, legs, arms, and shoulders
• Stretches front of body
• Strengthens core muscles

Caution
• Back issues
• Pregnancy

Annotation Key
Bold text indicates strengthening muscles
Black text indicates stretching muscles
* indicates deep muscles

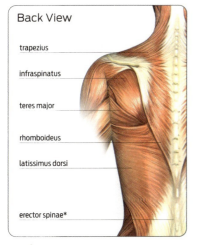

Back View
- trapezius
- infraspinatus
- teres major
- rhomboideus
- latissimus dorsi
- erector spinae*

- deltoideus posterior
- gluteus medius*
- gluteus maximus

85

ANATOMY OF FITNESS • YOGA

Half-Frog Pose
(Ardha Bhekasana)

Half-Frog Pose is great preparation for Bow Pose (pages 88–89). It helps to stretch the muscles that will be used in the full expression of the pose.

1 Lie on your stomach. Prop yourself up onto your forearms with your elbows directly beneath your shoulders. (This is called Sphinx Pose.)

2 Bend your left knee, bringing your heel toward your left buttock. Reach your left arm behind you and grasp the outside of your foot as you continue to press the foot toward your left hip.

3 Continue to bring your left foot toward your left hip. Press your right forearm and elbow down into the floor to avoid collapsing into your left shoulder. Square your shoulders toward the front of your mat. Hold for 1 to 5 breaths. Repeat on the other side.

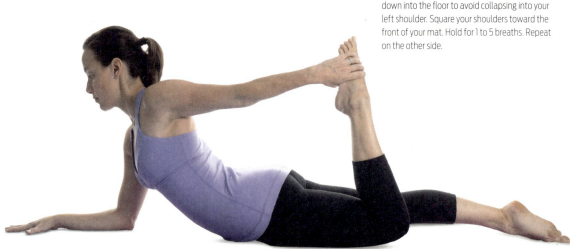

Correct form
· Engage your stomach muscles.

Avoid
· Sinking into your supporting shoulder.
· Twisting your neck.

Half-Frog Pose • BACKBENDS

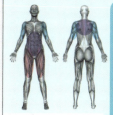

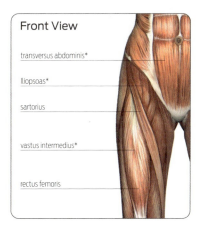

Front View

- transversus abdominis*
- Iliopsoas*
- sartorius
- vastus intermedius*
- rectus femoris

Annotation Key
Bold text indicates strengthening muscles
Black text indicates stretching muscles
* indicates deep muscles

Level
• Beginner

Duration
• 1–5 breaths

Benefits
• Stretches shoulders, torso, throat, abdomen, thighs, psoas, and ankles
• Strengthens back muscles
• Improves posture

Caution
• Lower-back issues
• Shoulder issues

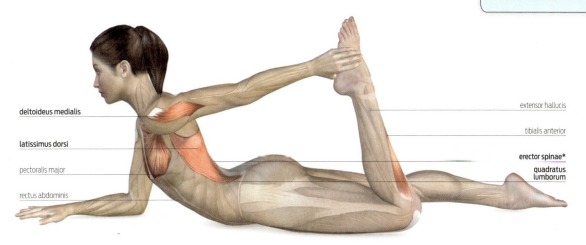

- **deltoideus medialis**
- **latissimus dorsi**
- pectoralis major
- rectus abdominis
- extensor hallucis
- tibialis anterior
- erector spinae*
- **quadratus lumborum**

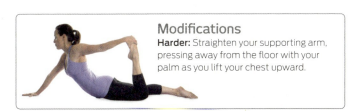

Modifications
Harder: Straighten your supporting arm, pressing away from the floor with your palm as you lift your chest upward.

87

Bow Pose

(Dhanurasana)

Bow Pose is sometimes referred to as "bow and arrow." *Dhanur* means bow-shaped, bent, or curved. This pose creates the shape of a bow ready to shoot an arrow.

1 Lie your stomach, with your forehead on the floor and your arms and legs extended straight behind you. Ground your pelvis and lower abdomen into the floor: this is your foundation.

2 Keep your legs hip-distance apart and bend both knees at the same time so that your ankles and shins are in line over your knees.

3 Inhaling, reach your arms back and grab your ankles with your right hand wrapping around the outside of the right foot and the left hand wrapping around the outside of the left foot.

4 Keep your arms straight as you exhale to lift your chest and thighs away from the floor. Pull your feet away from your head to help lift your chest higher.

5 Find internal rotation in both thighs, allowing your inner thighs to move up toward the ceiling. Draw your tailbone slightly downward to alleviate crunching in your lower back. Balance on your navel to find equal extension between the lift of your chest and that of your legs. Hold for 3 to 5 breaths.

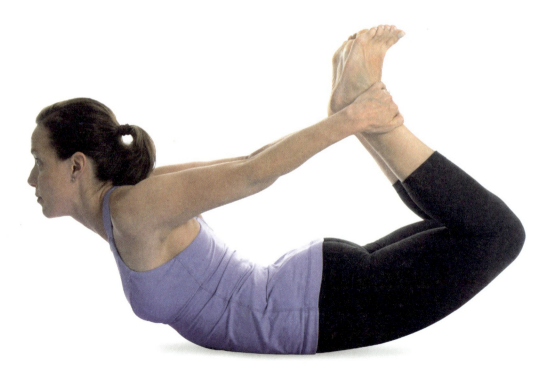

Bow Pose • **BACKBENDS**

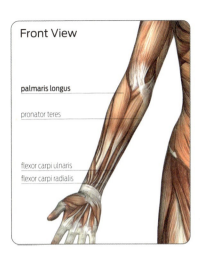

Front View

palmaris longus

pronator teres

flexor carpi ulnaris
flexor carpi radialis

Correct form
- Lengthen your tailbone to create space for your lower back.
- Squeeze your shoulder blades toward each other to help lift your chest.
- Lift your chest and thighs simultaneously.

Avoid
- Allowing your thighs to externally rotate.

Annotation Key
Bold text indicates strengthening muscles
Black text indicates stretching muscles
* indicates deep muscles

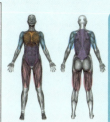

Level
- Intermediate

Duration
- 3–5 breaths

Benefits
- Stretches shoulders, chest, abdomen, and thighs
- Strengthens spine
- Aids digestion
- Massages the abdominal organs

Caution
- Lower-back issues
- Knee pain
- Shoulder issues
- Pregnancy

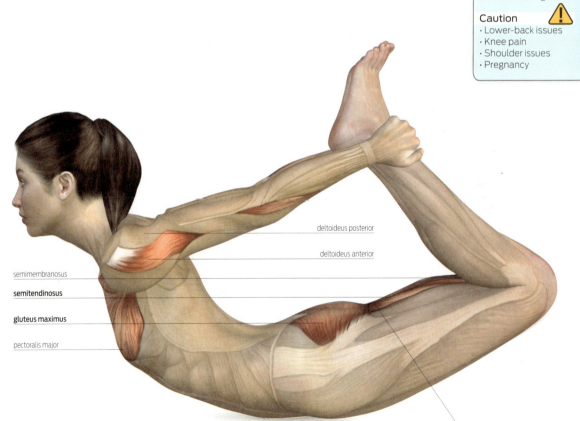

deltoideus posterior
deltoideus anterior

semimembranosus
semitendinosus
gluteus maximus
pectoralis major

adductor magnus

ANATOMY OF FITNESS • YOGA

Bridge Pose
(Setu Bandha Sarvangasana)

Although effective as preparation for Wheel Pose (pages 92–93), Bridge Pose is also very restorative when practiced on its own.

1 Lie on your back. Bend your knees so that they are directly over your ankles. Your feet should be hip-width apart and parallel. Extend your arms along your sides with the palms facing up.

2 Keep the back of your head, your shoulders, and your upper back on the floor as you press your heels down and lift your hips up. Draw your tailbone down toward your knees to lengthen your lower back.

3 Roll your shoulders underneath you one at a time, externally rotating your outer, upper arms to open your upper back. Draw your shoulders blades in toward your chest as you broaden across your collarbones. Bring your chest toward your chin, lifting the chin to make space for the back of your neck. Keep the natural curve of your cervical spine.

4 Find resistance between your knees so that they don't open too wide. Keep your feet firmly planted with the arches lifting. Roll your inner thighs down toward the floor. Aim to hold for 5 breaths.

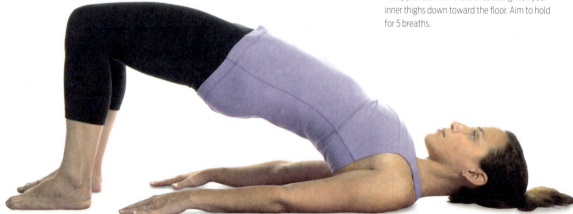

Correct form
- Focus on bending your upper back and chest.
- If desired, try placing a block beneath your sacrum to support your back.
- Keep your legs active by contracting your hamstrings.

Avoid
- Sticking out your stomach or ribs.
- Bending from your lower back.
- Clenching your buttocks together.

Bridge Pose • **BACKBENDS**

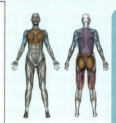

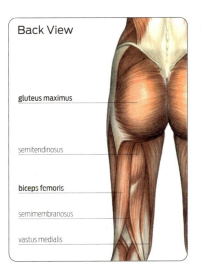

Back View

gluteus maximus

semitendinosus

biceps femoris

semimembranosus

vastus medialis

Annotation Key
Bold text indicates strengthening muscles
Black text indicates stretching muscles
* indicates deep muscles

Level
• Beginner

Duration
• 5 breaths

Benefits
• Stretches neck, chest, spine, and hip flexors
• Calms mind and body
• Strengthens legs, especially quadriceps, and rhomboids
• Opens pectorals, deltoids, and intercostals
• Releases tension in upper and lower-back

Caution
• Knee issues
• Lower-back issues
• Neck issues

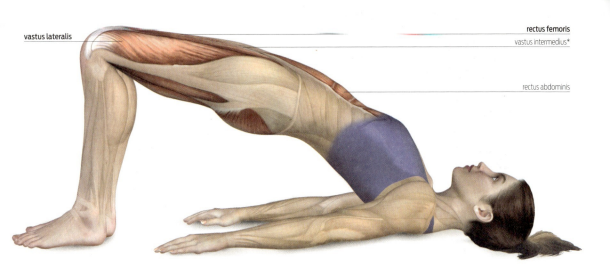

vastus lateralis

rectus femoris
vastus intermedius*

rectus abdominis

91

ANATOMY OF FITNESS • YOGA

Wheel Pose
(Urdhva Dhanurasana)

Highly invigorating and energizing, Wheel Pose is a deep, challenging backbend.

Correct form
- Keep your feet parallel, even as you transition into and out of the pose.
- After lifting onto the crown of your head, squeeze your elbows toward each other to keep your elbows over your wrists.
- While holding the pose, draw your tailbone down toward your knees and lift your frontal hipbones up toward your ribs.

Avoid
- Avoid letting your thighs externally rotate, as this can cause compression in your lower back.

1 Lie on your back, with your knees bent and your feet hip-width apart. Inhale your arms straight up to the ceiling with your palms facing away from you. Then, bend your arms and place your hands on the floor next to your ears, shoulder-width apart, with your fingers facing the same direction as your toes.

2 Press your hands and feet into the floor as you lift your hips up as if you were coming into Bridge Pose (pages 90–91).

3 Lift onto the crown of your head. Pause and press your palms into the floor, spreading your fingers wide and grounding down through every knuckle and through the base of your thumb and index finger.

4 Straighten your arms, and wrap your outer, upper arms inward to find external rotation. Press down through all four corners of your feet, shifting your weight onto your heels. Roll your inner thighs toward the floor as you firm your outer hips inward. Let your head fall between your shoulders in a comfortable position. Hold for 3 to 5 breaths.

5 To come out of the pose, bend your arms and shift your body weight toward your shoulders as you slowly descend, landing on the back of your head and your shoulder blades.

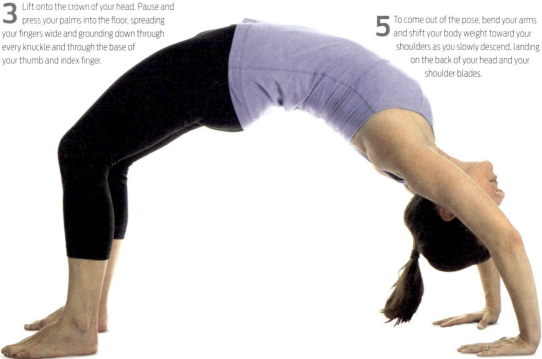

Wheel Pose • **BACKBENDS**

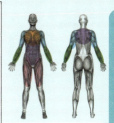

Back View

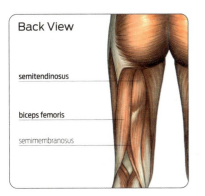

- semitendinosus
- biceps femoris
- semimembranosus

Annotation Key
Bold text indicates strengthening muscles
Black text indicates stretching muscles
* indicates deep muscles

Level
• Intermediate/Advanced

Duration
• 3–5 breaths

Benefits
• Stretches inner organs, opening up lungs
• Increases flexibility in spine
• Improves posture
• Builds stamina and strength
• Energizes and invigorates, counteracting depression

Caution
• Elbow issues
• Knee issues
• Lower-back issues
• Neck issues
• SI joint issues
• Wrist issues
• Pregnancy

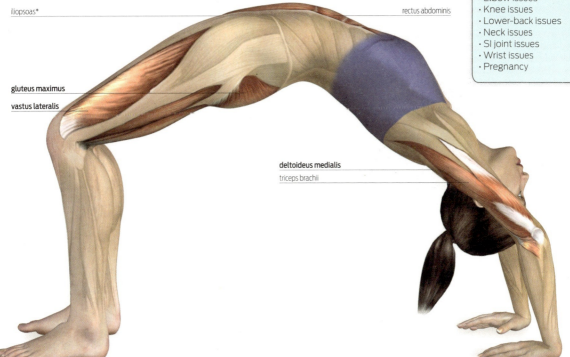

- iliopsoas*
- rectus abdominis
- gluteus maximus
- vastus lateralis
- deltoideus medialis
- triceps brachii

93

ANATOMY OF FITNESS • YOGA

Camel Pose
(Ustrasana)

Camel Pose is a heart-opening backbend that stretches the shoulders and lower back.

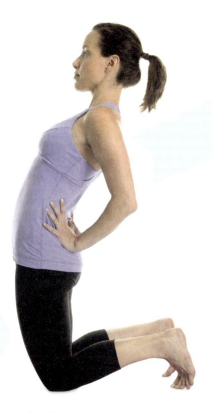

1 Kneel on your mat, with your knees hip-width apart and shins and feet aligned behind them. The tops of your feet should be on the floor, your toes pointing straight back.

2 Bend your elbows, and bring your hands to your lower back, fingers pointing upward. Draw your elbows together, opening your chest, internally rotate your thighs, and use the heels of your palms to draw your buttocks toward the floor as you lift out of your lower back.

3 Bend from your upper back, and straighten your arms as you reach behind you to grasp your heels. Keep your hips directly above your knees; if your hips shift backward as you reach for your toes, keep your hands on your lower back. With practice, you will eventually be able to bend back to reach your heels.

4 Broaden across your collarbones and press your shoulder blades in and up to open your chest and shoulders. Allow your head to drop back. Hold for 1 to 5 breaths.

5 To come out of the pose, exhale to lift your head and torso and sit into Child's Pose (pages 146–147).

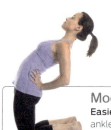

Modifications
Easier: Instead of reaching for your ankles, place your hands on the sides of your lower back.

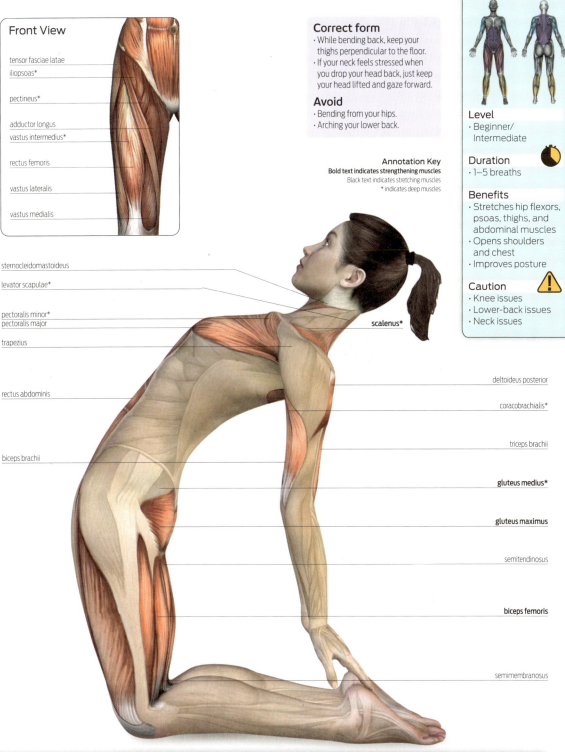

ANATOMY OF FITNESS • YOGA

Fish Pose
(Matsyasana)

Fish Pose is often practiced as a counter pose to Shoulder Stand (pages 120–121).

1 Lie on your back with your legs bent, feet on the floor. Place your hands slightly underneath your buttocks and begin to lift your hips off the floor.

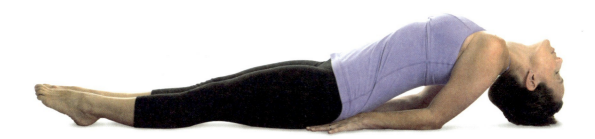

2 Pressing your palms, elbows, and forearms into the floor and drawing your shoulder blades together, lift your head and chest off the floor.

3 With the top of your head on the floor, extend your legs straight onto your mat. Internally rotate your thighs and press them downward. Reach out through the balls of your feet as you hold for 3 to 5 breaths.

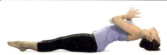

Modifications
Harder: Instead of resting your lower arms and hands along the floor, position your upper arms parallel to the floor and your hands in front of your chest, palms together.

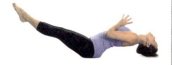

Harder: To make the pose even more challenging, keep your legs together and extended as you lift them off the ground—making sure that you maintain your form.

Fish Pose • **BACKBENDS**

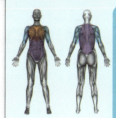

Level
- Beginner/Intermediate

Duration
- 3–5 breaths

Benefits
- Opens chest
- Relieves tightness in upper back and throat
- Stretches hip flexors (psoas) and muscles between the ribs (intercostals)
- Improves posture

Caution
- Lower-back issues
- Neck issues

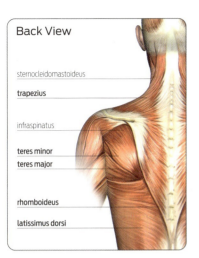

Back View
- sternocleidomastoideus
- **trapezius**
- infraspinatus
- teres minor
- teres major
- rhomboideus
- latissimus dorsi

Correct form
- As you hold, engage your stomach muscles to support your lower back.

Avoid
- Sinking into your lower back.

Annotation Key
Bold text indicates strengthening muscles
Black text indicates stretching muscles
* indicates deep muscles

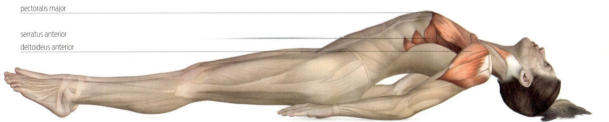

- pectoralis major
- serratus anterior
- deltoideus anterior

Modifications
Easier: Try placing one block underneath your thoracic spine and another beneath your head, making Fish Pose into a restorative backbend.

97

ANATOMY OF FITNESS • YOGA

Pigeon Pose
(Eka Pada Rajakapotsana)

Pigeon Pose is especially challenging because it demands flexibility in the hips, thighs, spine, and shoulders.

1 From Downward-Facing Dog (pages 116–117), inhale and lift your right leg up behind you.

2 On an exhale, bend your right knee into your chest and then lower your body so that your right knee is on the floor in front of you, foot facing left, right shin and foot on the floor. Draw your right shin slightly forward, and flex your right ankle to keep your knee in alignment.

3 Extend your left leg behind you, with the top of your foot on the floor and toes pointing straight back.

4 Slowly lift your torso upright, bend your left knee, and hold onto your foot with your left hand. Lift up out of your lower back by drawing your tailbone down as you lift your public bone toward your frontal hipbones.

5 Bring your foot into the crook of your left elbow before reaching your right arm up, bending the elbow toward the ceiling, and clasping your hands as you continue to square your hips and shoulders. Hold for 1 to 5 breaths. Repeat on the other side.

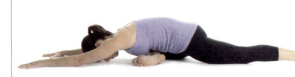

Modifications
Easier: Try making the pose more restorative by "walking" your hands in front of you and releasing your torso into a forward bend. Place your forehead on the floor and hold for several breaths.

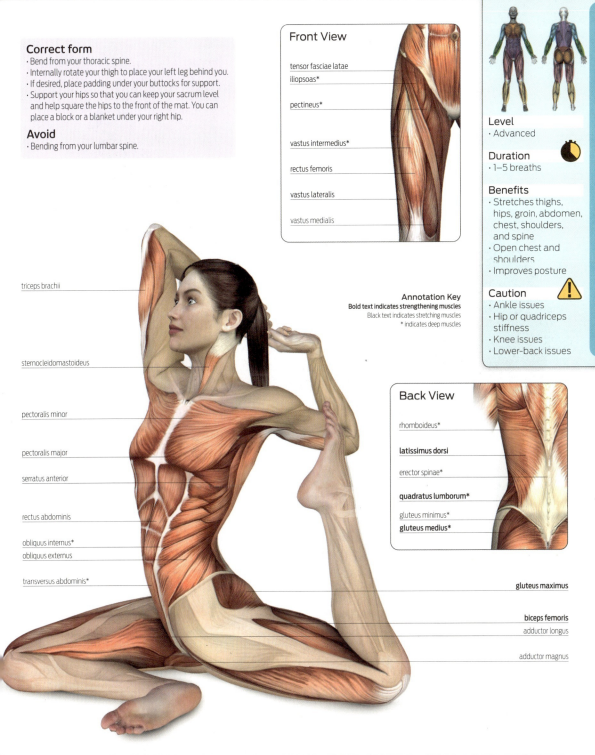

ANATOMY OF FITNESS • YOGA

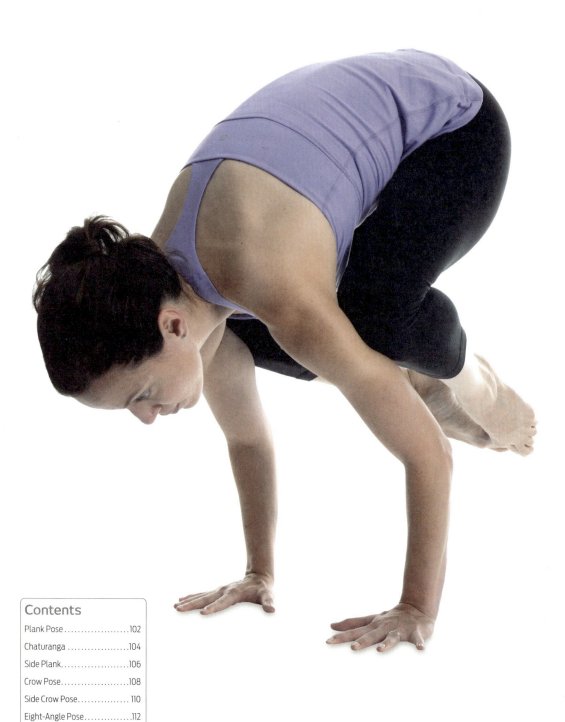

Contents

Plank Pose	102
Chaturanga	104
Side Plank	106
Crow Pose	108
Side Crow Pose	110
Eight-Angle Pose	112

ARM SUPPORTS

Arm Supports range from a classic Plank Pose to an intricate and advanced arm balance. All require a combination of strength and flexibility; one might be strong enough to do the pose, but not open enough in the hips or shoulders to carry it out correctly, or vice versa. Arm Supports take time and practice. By repeating them often, you will see results.

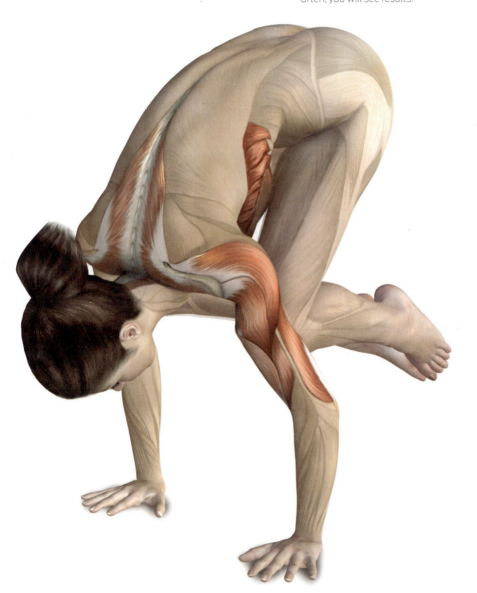

Plank Pose

Plank Pose plays a role in many yoga sequences, including the Sun Salutations. However, it can also be practiced on its own. Once you master the basic pose, challenge yourself by holding it for 30 seconds, 1 minute, or eventually even 2 or 3 minutes. Remember to keep breathing!

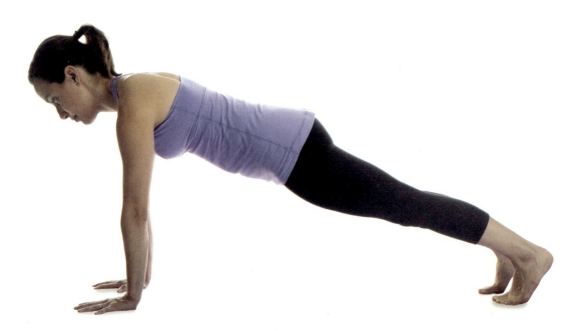

1 From Downward-Facing Dog (pages 116–117), inhale and shift your weight forward so that your shoulders are in line with your wrists. At the same time, come onto the balls of your feet, with your toes spread out and your heels reaching back.

2 Keep your arms straight and parallel to each other, externally rotating your outer upper arms so that your inner elbows draw forward.

3 As you hold the pose, soften between your shoulder blades and melt your heart down as you broaden across your collarbones to lift your sternum. Internally rotate your inner thighs, keeping the thighs firm. Lengthen your tailbone down toward your heels. Hold for 1 to 5 breaths.

Plank Pose • ARM SUPPORTS

Annotation Key
Bold text indicates strengthening muscles
Black text indicates stretching muscles
* indicates deep muscles

Level
• Beginner

Duration
• 1–5 breaths

Benefits
• Strengthens arms and core muscles

Caution
• Wrist issues

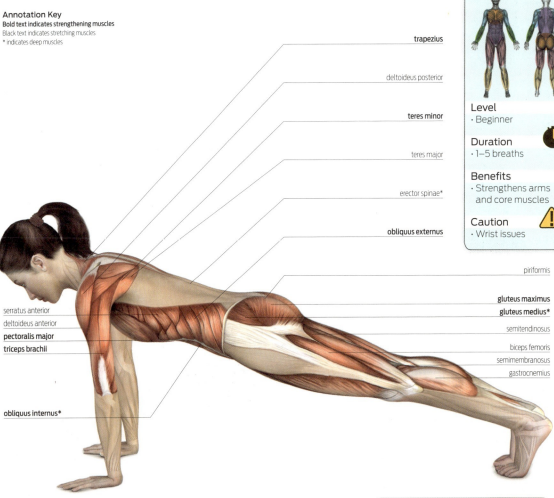

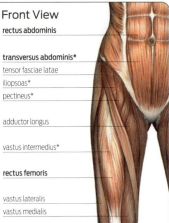

Correct form
• Make sure your wrist creases are parallel to the front of the mat.
• Spread your fingers wide, and ground down through every knuckle.
• Use your breath to get you through holding the pose.

Avoid
• Lifting your fingers off the floor.
• Rounding your upper back.

ANATOMY OF FITNESS • YOGA

Chaturanga
(Chaturanga Dandasana)

Chaturanga, sometimes called Four-Limbed Staff Pose, challenges your core strength and stability. It is also an effective strengthener for the arms, legs, and shoulders.

1 Begin in Plank Pose (pages 102–103), with your hands planted on the floor shoulder distance apart, your arms straight and your body lifted off the mat to form a straight line. Your feet should be parallel, with heels lifted. Exhale as you bend your elbows over your wrists and lower yourself down so that your shoulders are in line with your elbows. As you lower, ground your palm and fingers down into the floor. The thumb and index finger have a tendency to want to lift up, so make a special effort to press down between the two.

2 Hold the pose, rotating your inner thighs and drawing your tailbone downward so that you don't sink into your lower back. Lift your thighs away from the floor. Draw your shoulder blades together as you lift the heads of the shoulders away from the floor. Take 1 to 2 full breaths.

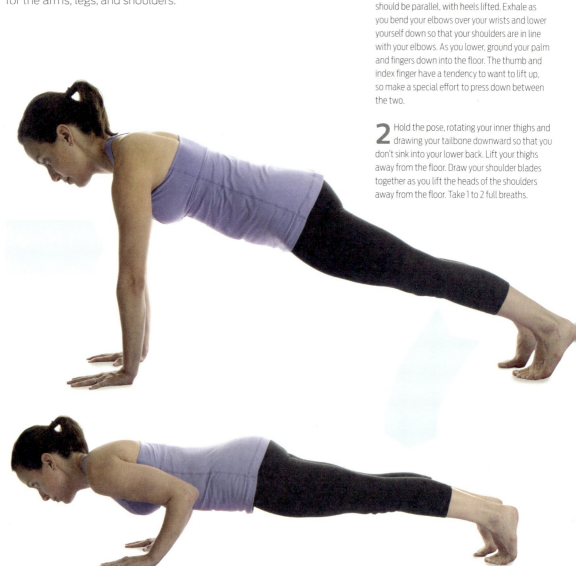

Chaturanga • ARM SUPPORTS

Front View

- obliquus internus*
- **rectus abdominis**
- obliquus externus
- **transversus abdominis***
- tensor fasciae latae
- iliopsoas*
- pectineus*
- adductor longus
- vastus intermedius*
- **rectus femoris**
- vastus medialis
- vastus lateralis

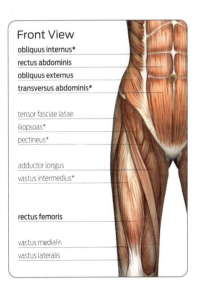

Back View

- semitendinosus
- biceps femoris
- semimembranosus
- soleus

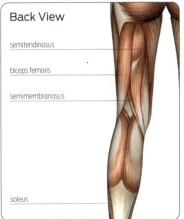

Correct form
- Keep the back of your neck long by gazing slightly beyond the edge of your mat.

Avoid
- Bending your elbows so much that your chest collapses and your shoulders round forward.
- Dropping your hips lower than your shoulders.

Back View

- trapezius
- deltoideus medialis
- **infraspinatus***
- **supraspinatus***
- **subscapularis***
- teres major
- rhomboideus*

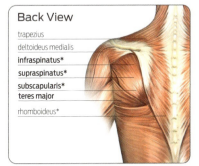

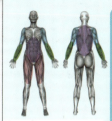

Level
- Intermediate

Duration
- 1–2 breaths

Benefits
- Strengthens spine, abdomen, arms, and wrists

Caution
- Shoulder issues
- Wrist issues
- Pregnancy

Annotation Key
Bold text indicates strengthening muscles
Black text indicates stretching muscles
* indicates deep muscles

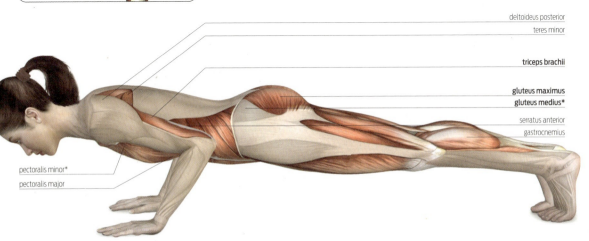

- pectoralis minor*
- pectoralis major
- **deltoideus posterior**
- **teres minor**
- **triceps brachii**
- **gluteus maximus**
- **gluteus medius***
- serratus anterior
- gastrocnemius

105

ANATOMY OF FITNESS • YOGA

Side Plank
(Vasisthasana)

The challenge of Side Plank Pose lies in maintaining alignment in your spine and legs. Here gravity works against you; try not to let your spine twist, your hips fall forward or lift too high, or your pelvis sink toward the floor. Over time, this will become easier.

Correct form
- Elongate your arms and legs as much as possible.
- Keep your feet stacked and flexed.

Avoid
- Letting your spine or legs fall out of alignment.

1 Begin in Plank Pose (pages 102–103), with your hands planted on the floor shoulder distance apart, your arms straight and your body lifted off the mat to form a straight line. Your feet should be parallel, with heels lifted. Shift your weight toward the right side of your body, pivoting to the outside edge of your right foot, and stack your left foot on top of your right.

2 On an exhalation, bring your left arm up so that it is perpendicular to the floor. Elongate your body, aiming to form a straight line from head to heels. Turn your head to gaze up toward your left hand.

3 Maintain your balance as you press your right palm into the floor. Hold for 3 to 5 breaths. Repeat on the other side.

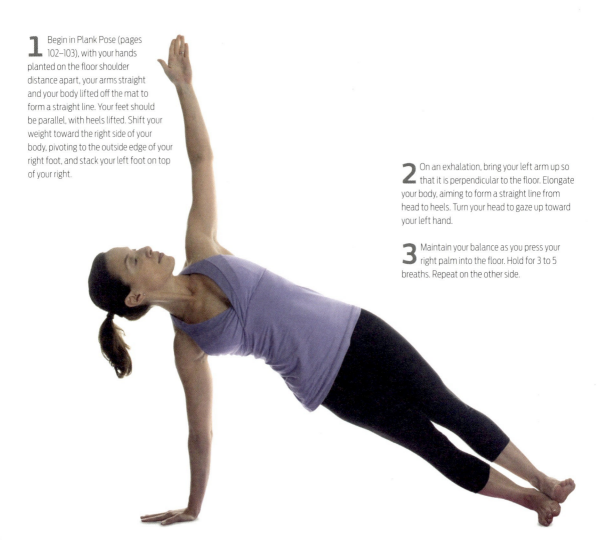

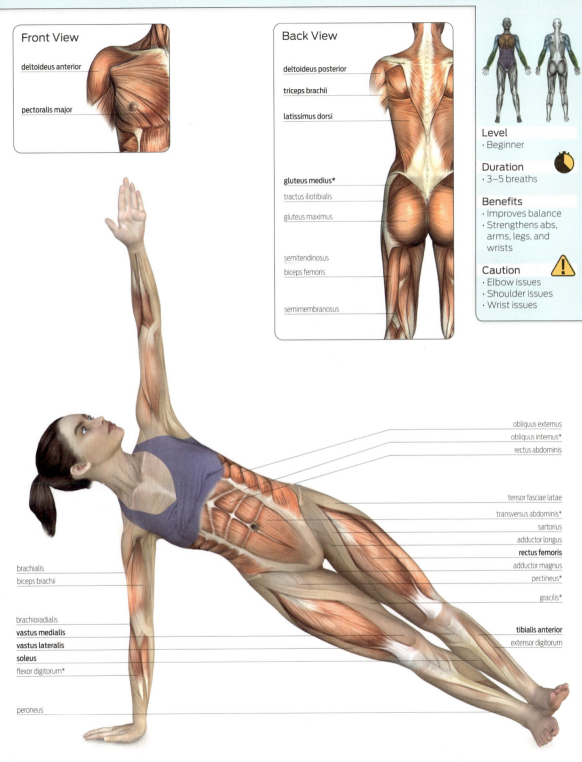

ANATOMY OF FITNESS • YOGA

Crow Pose
(Bakasana)

Crow Pose is an exciting arm balance. As you perform this pose you will encounter the fear of falling, which you will eventually overcome.

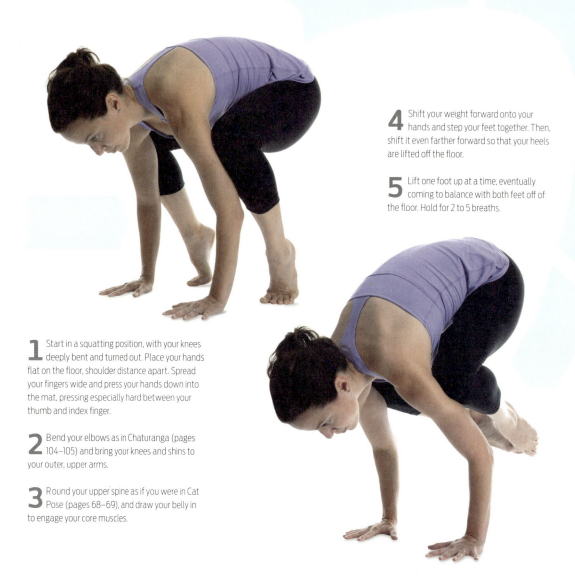

1 Start in a squatting position, with your knees deeply bent and turned out. Place your hands flat on the floor, shoulder distance apart. Spread your fingers wide and press your hands down into the mat, pressing especially hard between your thumb and index finger.

2 Bend your elbows as in Chaturanga (pages 104–105) and bring your knees and shins to your outer, upper arms.

3 Round your upper spine as if you were in Cat Pose (pages 68–69), and draw your belly in to engage your core muscles.

4 Shift your weight forward onto your hands and step your feet together. Then, shift it even farther forward so that your heels are lifted off the floor.

5 Lift one foot up at a time, eventually coming to balance with both feet off of the floor. Hold for 2 to 5 breaths.

Crow Pose • ARM SUPPORTS

Correct form
- Make sure that your wrist creases line up with the front edge of your mat.
- Keep your hands pressed into the floor.
- Allow yourself to gaze slightly forward, as this will help you to balance.
- Place a blanket in front of you if you fear falling forward.

Avoid
- Dropping your head, as this may cause you to tip forward.
- Lifting or twisting your neck to the point where it feels strained.

Level
- Intermediate/Advanced

Duration
- 2–5 breaths

Benefits
- Strengthens arms, wrists, and core
- Stretches spine
- Improves balance

Caution
- Wrist issues
- Shoulder issues

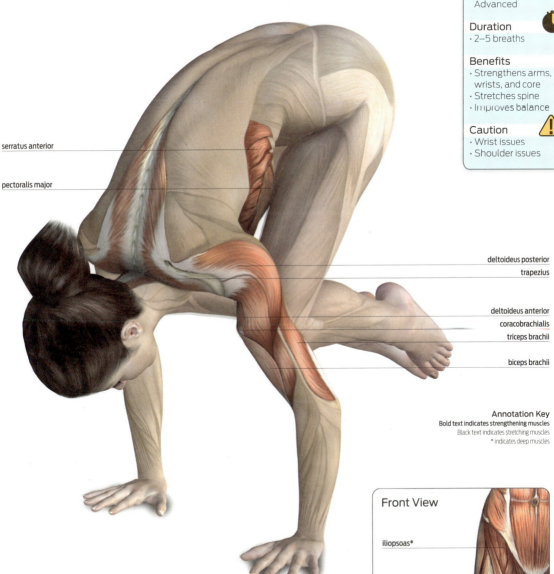

serratus anterior
pectoralis major
deltoideus posterior
trapezius
deltoideus anterior
coracobrachialis
triceps brachii
biceps brachii

Annotation Key
Bold text indicates strengthening muscles
Black text indicates stretching muscles
* indicates deep muscles

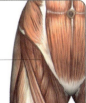

Front View

iliopsoas*

ANATOMY OF FITNESS • YOGA

Side Crow Pose
(Parsva Bakasana)

Poses like this difficult arm balance remind us that yoga takes practice. Be patient—and playful!

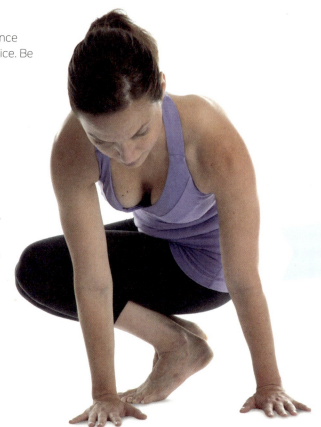

1 Start in a squatting position, with your knees deeply bent, your thighs parallel to the floor, and your feet together.

2 Begin to twist your entire torso to the left, placing your right elbow at the outside of your right thigh. Deepen the twist, bringing the right side of your body, including the ribs, to the left. Come onto the balls of your feet, allowing your heels and hips to lift as you place both hands onto the floor, shoulder distance apart. Spread your fingers wide and ground down through every knuckle, especially between the thumb and index fingers.

3 Shift your weight forward onto your hands and bend your arms as in Chaturanga (pages 104–105), bringing your elbows back. Think of drawing your elbows toward each other to find resistance. Press your right elbow into your left outer hip as you rest your outer left thigh on your right upper arm, using your right arm as if it were a shelf.

Correct form
- Draw your stomach in to activate your core muscles.
- If desired, place a block beneath your forehead.
- Keep your chest lifted as you shift your weight forward.
- While balancing, keep your hips, knees, ankles, and feet stacked directly above each other.

Avoid
- Letting a fear of falling over jeopardize your balance as you look forward.

Side Crow Pose • **ARM SUPPORTS**

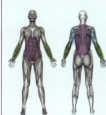

4 Continue to shift your weight forward, lifting your feet off the floor either one by one or simultaneously. Find your balance and hold for 3 to 5 breaths. Repeat on the other side.

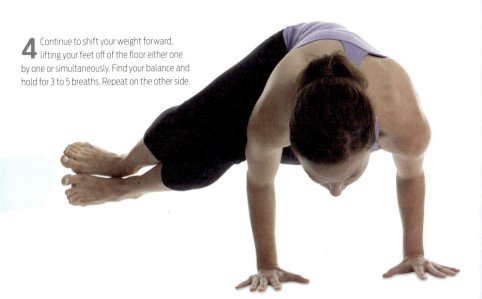

Level
• Advanced

Duration
• 3–5 breaths

Benefits
• Aids digestion
• Strengthens forearms and wrists
• Stretches spine
• Improves balance

Caution
• Elbow issues
• Lower-back issues
• Shoulder issues
• Wrist issues
• Pregnancy

Annotation Key
Bold text indicates strengthening muscles
Black text indicates stretching muscles
* indicates deep muscles

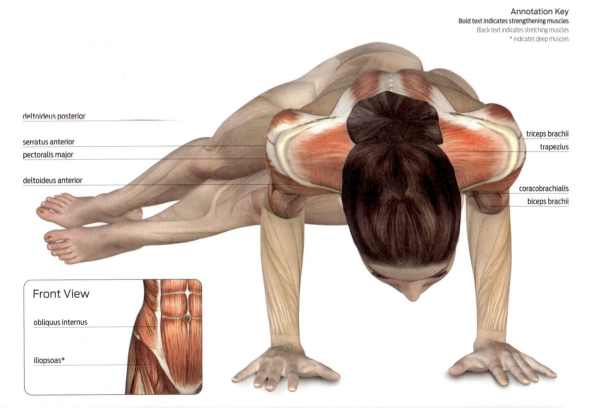

deltoideus posterior
serratus anterior
pectoralis major
deltoideus anterior

triceps brachii
trapezius
coracobrachialis
biceps brachii

Front View
obliquus internus
iliopsoas*

111

Eight-Angle Pose
(Astavakrasana)

Eight-Angle Pose can seem intimidating at first. Take it step by step; eventually, with patient practice, you will be able to carry out the full pose.

1. Sit with both legs extended in front of you and your hands on the floor at your sides. Bend your right knee so that the foot is flat on the floor, and bend your left leg so that the knee is out to the side and the foot is pointed toward your groin.

2. Lift your right foot and shin upward, parallel to the floor, placing the right foot into the left elbow crease. Open your right knee out to the side and bring the knee to the inside of the right elbow, cradling your leg. You can spend several breaths here to open the hip.

3. Bring your right hand underneath your right shin or calf and bend forward slightly to bring your right knee over your right shoulder. Try to get the leg as high up on your shoulder as you can.

4. Keep your right leg bent over your right shoulder as your press both hands flat against the floor. Then, lift your left leg up off the floor and cross your left ankle over your right ankle.

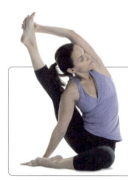

Modifications
Easier: Instead of balancing your body weight on your arms after twisting to the side, bend one leg and rest it on the floor in front of you. Extend the other leg and grasp the foot with your opposite hand. Turn your gaze away from your lifted leg and hold. This is called Compass Pose.

Eight-Angle Pose • **ARM SUPPORTS**

5 Lift your hips up and hinge your torso forward parallel to the floor as you bend your elbows as in Chaturanga (pages 104–105). Keep your ankles crossed as you straighten your legs out to the right. Hold for 1 to 5 breaths. Repeat on the other side.

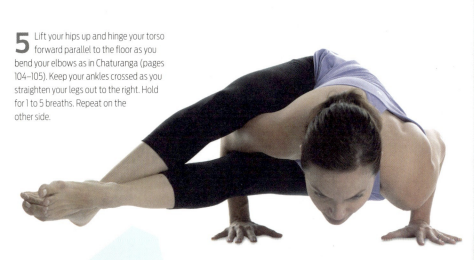

Level
• Advanced

Duration
• 1–5 breaths

Benefits
• Strengthens arms and wrists
• Stretches hamstrings, hips, and shoulders
• Tones abdomen

Caution
• Elbow issues
• Shoulder issues
• Wrist issues

Annotation Key
Bold text indicates strengthening muscles
Black text indicates stretching muscles
* indicates deep muscles

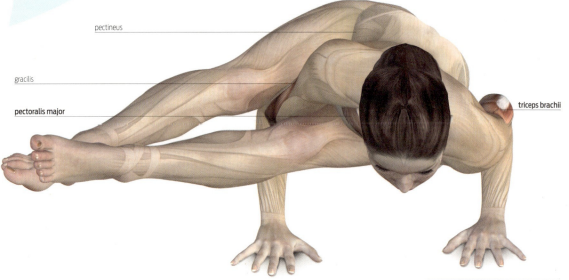

pectineus

gracilis

pectoralis major

triceps brachii

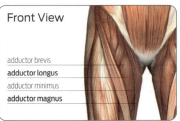

Front View

adductor brevis
adductor longus
adductor minimus
adductor magnus

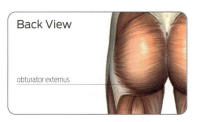

Back View

obturator externus

Correct form
• Allow yourself to stop at any step until you are ready for the full pose.
• Press your hands down into the floor to help lift your hips and legs.
• Gaze forward.

Avoid
• Forcing your shoulder into position, as this could cause strain or injury.

ANATOMY OF FITNESS • YOGA

Contents
- Downward-Facing Dog........ 116
- Plow Pose..................... 118
- Shoulder Stand 120
- Head Stand 122

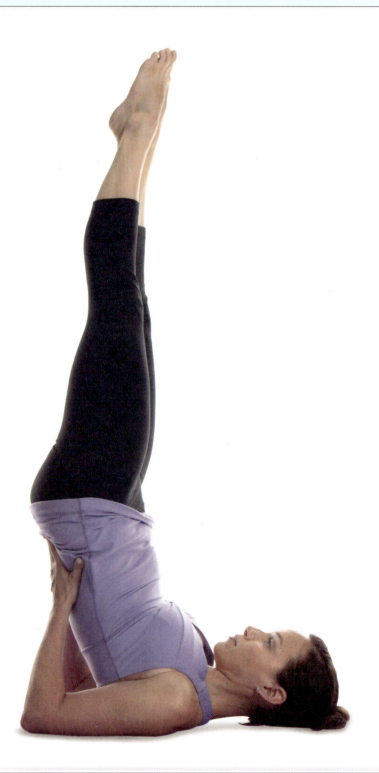

Inverted Poses

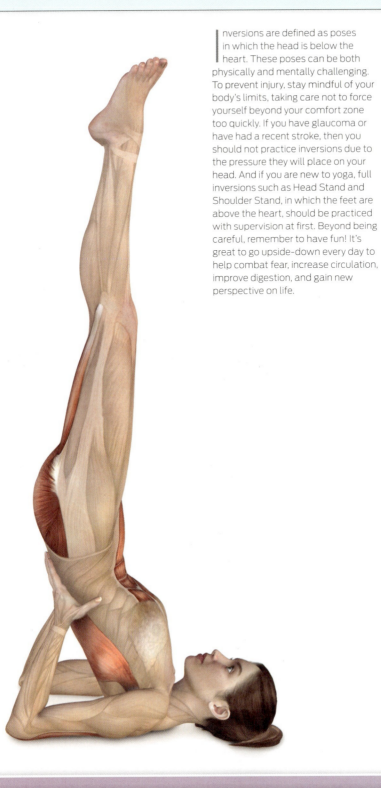

Inversions are defined as poses in which the head is below the heart. These poses can be both physically and mentally challenging. To prevent injury, stay mindful of your body's limits, taking care not to force yourself beyond your comfort zone too quickly. If you have glaucoma or have had a recent stroke, then you should not practice inversions due to the pressure they will place on your head. And if you are new to yoga, full inversions such as Head Stand and Shoulder Stand, in which the feet are above the heart, should be practiced with supervision at first. Beyond being careful, remember to have fun! It's great to go upside-down every day to help combat fear, increase circulation, improve digestion, and gain new perspective on life.

Downward-Facing Dog
(Adho Mukha Svanasana)

Downward-Facing Dog is among the most frequently performed yoga poses—one you'll come into time and again. "Down Dog," as it is often known, stretches and strengthens the entire body.

1 Begin on your hands and knees, with your hands aligned under your shoulders and your knees under your hips.

2 Tuck your toes under, and "walk" your hands forward about a palm's distance in front of your shoulders. With hands and toes planted, lift your hips up as you straighten your legs and draw your heels toward the floor.

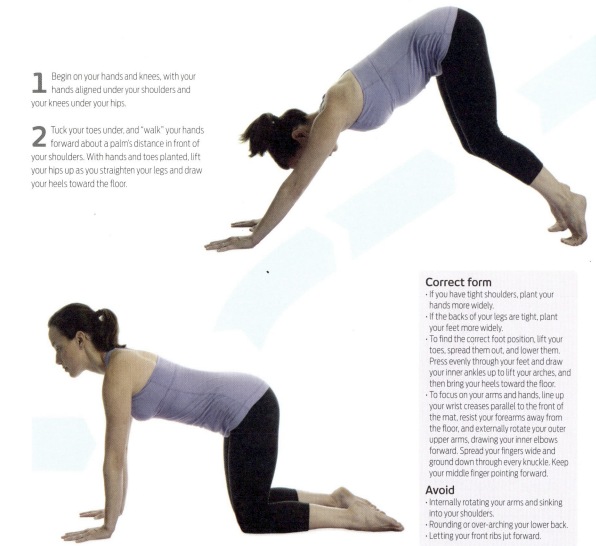

Correct form
- If you have tight shoulders, plant your hands more widely.
- If the backs of your legs are tight, plant your feet more widely.
- To find the correct foot position, lift your toes, spread them out, and lower them. Press evenly through your feet and draw your inner ankles up to lift your arches, and then bring your heels toward the floor.
- To focus on your arms and hands, line up your wrist creases parallel to the front of the mat, resist your forearms away from the floor, and externally rotate your outer upper arms, drawing your inner elbows forward. Spread your fingers wide and ground down through every knuckle. Keep your middle finger pointing forward.

Avoid
- Internally rotating your arms and sinking into your shoulders.
- Rounding or over-arching your lower back.
- Letting your front ribs jut forward.

Downward-Facing Dog • **INVERTED POSES**

3 Press your chest toward your thighs, and bring your head between your arms. Lengthen up through your tailbone and keep your thighs slightly internally rotated, finding a neutral pelvis. Gaze between your feet or toward your navel. Aim to hold for at least 5 to 10 breaths.

Level
- Beginner

Duration
- 5–10 breaths or longer

Benefits
- Strengthens arms and legs
- Stretches spine, hamstrings, calves, and arches of feet
- Aids digestion
- Helps to relieve menstrual cramps
- Helps to relieve headache

Caution
- Low blood pressure
- Shoulder injury
- Torn hamstring

Annotation Key
Bold text indicates strengthening muscles
Black text indicates stretching muscles
* indicates deep muscles

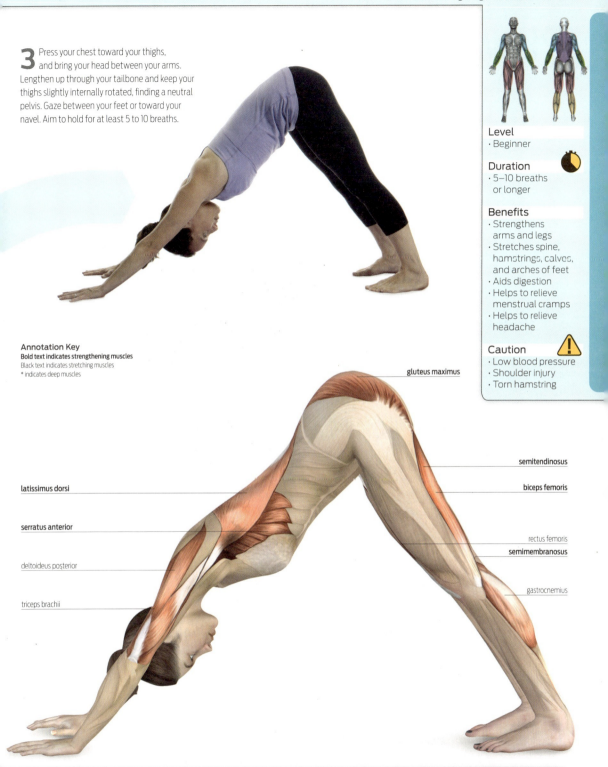

117

ANATOMY OF FITNESS • YOGA

Plow Pose

(Halasana)

Usually practiced as a way to get into, or down from, Shoulder Stand, Plow Pose is also a great pose to hold on its own. Try staying in the pose for up to 5 minutes to help release tension in your upper back.

1 Lie on your back with your legs bent and your arms along your sides, palms flat on the floor. Tighten your ab muscles, and lift your knees off the floor, extending your legs straight upward. On an exhalation, press your arms into the floor, and lift your knees even higher so that your buttocks and hips come off the floor.

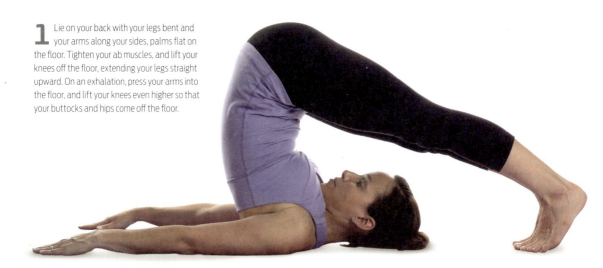

2 Roll your back off the mat as you continue to lift your knees toward your face, and bring your hips toward your shoulders.

3 On an inhalation, tuck your tailbone and straighten your legs back toward your head so that your torso is perpendicular to the floor. Exhaling, keep extending your legs beyond your head, aiming to touch the floor with your toes. Hold for 5 to 10 breaths, challenging yourself to stay in the position longer if possible.

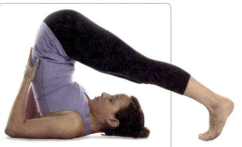

Modifications
Easier: Bend your arms at the elbows and use your hands to support your lower back.

Plow Pose • INVERTED POSES

Targeted Muscles

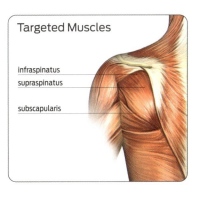

- infraspinatus
- supraspinatus
- subscapularis

Annotation Key
Bold text indicates strengthening muscles
Black text indicates stretching muscles
* indicates deep muscles

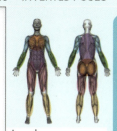

Level
• Beginner

Duration
• 5-10 breaths or longer

Benefits
• Stretches and strengthens hamstrings, groin, and spine

Caution
• Lower-back issues

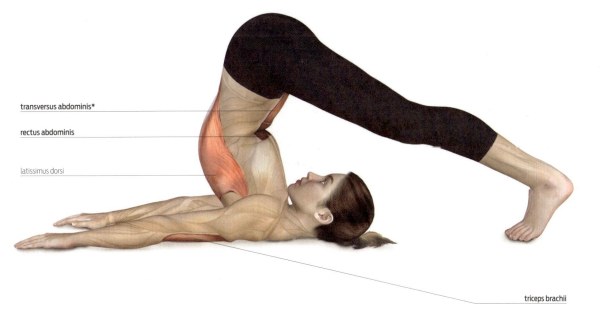

- transversus abdominis*
- rectus abdominis
- latissimus dorsi
- triceps brachii

Correct form
• Maintain a natural curve in your cervical spine, so that there is space beneath your neck.
• Externally rotate your shoulders.

Avoid
• Over-tucking your chin.
• Lifting your chin up high, which can cause neck strain.

119

ANATOMY OF FITNESS • YOGA

Shoulder Stand
(Sarvangasana)

Shoulder Stand is commonly referred to as the queen or mother of asanas.

1 Lie your back, with your arms extended along your sides. Bend your knees into your chest, and begin to curl your tailbone and hips off the floor as your roll your legs behind you into Plow Pose (pages 118–119). Extend your legs behind your head so that they are straight, with your toes tucked under.

2 Externally rotate your arms and roll your shoulders further beneath your back so that you can derive more support from your shoulders. Bend your elbows and draw them in toward each other, firming your shoulder blades. Place your palms onto your lower back, fingers pointing toward the ceiling.

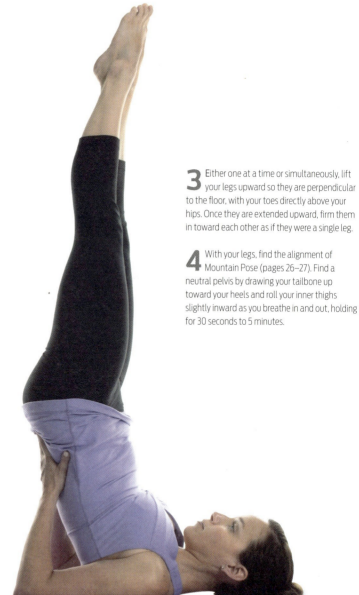

3 Either one at a time or simultaneously, lift your legs upward so they are perpendicular to the floor, with your toes directly above your hips. Once they are extended upward, firm them in toward each other as if they were a single leg.

4 With your legs, find the alignment of Mountain Pose (pages 26–27). Find a neutral pelvis by drawing your tailbone up toward your heels and roll your inner thighs slightly inward as you breathe in and out, holding for 30 seconds to 5 minutes.

Correct form
- Try placing blankets beneath your shoulders if the back of your neck feels strained.
- Keep your chin very slightly tucked.
- Keep a natural curve in your neck; you should be able to slide your hand in the space between your neck and the floor.
- Focus on a comfortable gazing point toward your belly button, or close your eyes.

Avoid
- Turning your head, which could injure your neck.
- Over-tucking your chin into your chest.

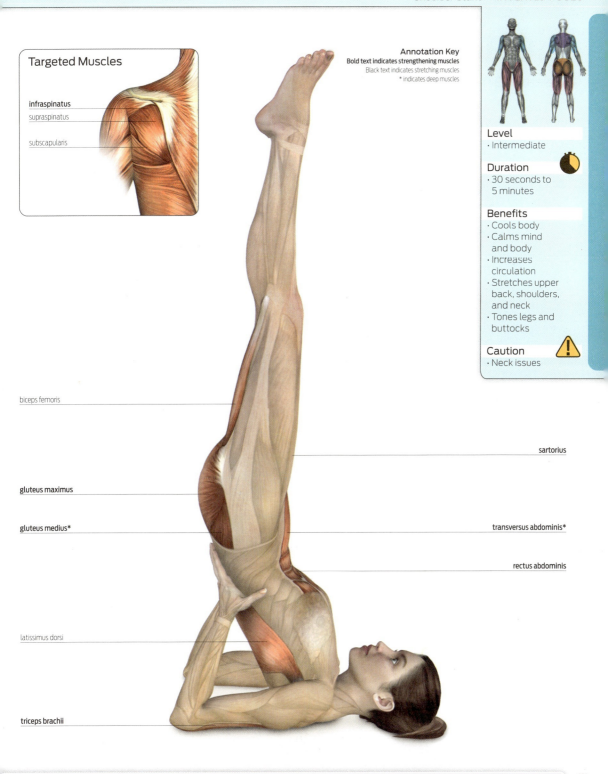

Head Stand

(Salamba Sirsasana)

Find clarity of mind through this heating inversion, which is often called the king of all yoga poses. If you are new to this pose, start by performing Head Stand against a wall. Once you feel more stable, you can come away from it until you are able to balance on your own.

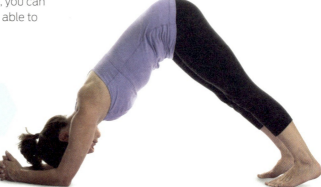

1 Place your mat against a wall, if desired. Come onto your hands and knees. Place your forearms on the floor, shoulder-width apart, externally rotating your outer, upper arms and interlacing your fingers. Tuck your toes under and lift your hips upward. This position is called Dolphin Pose. A great preparatory position for Head Stand, it can be held for 5 to 10 breaths.

2 Maintaining your alignment, slightly release the grip of your fingers so that your palms are more open while your fingers stay interlaced. Place the top of your head on the floor and the back of your head on your hands. Find a solid foundation, with your forearms and outer wrists pressing down.

3 Allowing your heels to lift off the floor, walk your feet toward your head until your hips are directly above your shoulders. At the same time, press your chest toward your thighs; this will help you to lift up into the full pose, helping to protect your neck from compression.

4 Bend one knee and then the other into your chest. Then, begin to straighten both legs up toward the ceiling. You can also place your feet against the wall before straightening them. Hold for as long as you can maintain your form.

5 Find a slight internal rotation in your thighs as you lengthen your tailbone up toward your heels. Reach the balls of your feet toward the ceiling to help activate the backs of your legs and your gluteal muscles. Try holding for 10 to 30 seconds, working up to 1 to 3 minutes.

Head Stand • **INVERTED POSES**

6 Come out of the pose by bending your knees into your chest and slowly lowering to the floor.

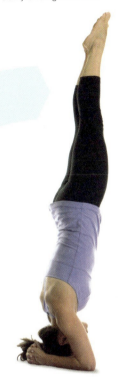

Annotation Key
Bold text indicates strengthening muscles
Black text indicates stretching muscles
* indicates deep muscles

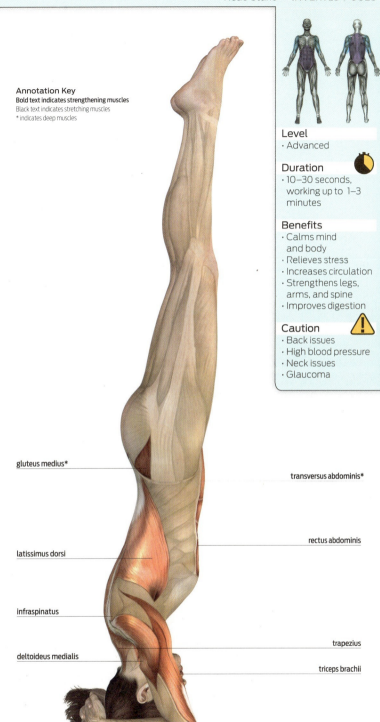

Level
• Advanced

Duration
• 10–30 seconds, working up to 1–3 minutes

Benefits
• Calms mind and body
• Relieves stress
• Increases circulation
• Strengthens legs, arms, and spine
• Improves digestion

Caution
• Back issues
• High blood pressure
• Neck issues
• Glaucoma

gluteus medius*

latissimus dorsi

infraspinatus

deltoideus medialis

transversus abdominis*

rectus abdominis

trapezius

triceps brachii

Correct form
• Press your forearms firmly and evenly into the floor.

Avoid
• Placing your forehead on the floor, as this can cause compression in your neck.

123

ANATOMY OF FITNESS • YOGA

Contents

Staff Pose	126
Easy Pose	128
Hero Pose	130
Cow-Face Pose	132
Full Lotus Pose	134
Full Boat Pose	136
Sage's Pose	138
Half Lord of the Fishes Pose	140
Monkey Pose	142

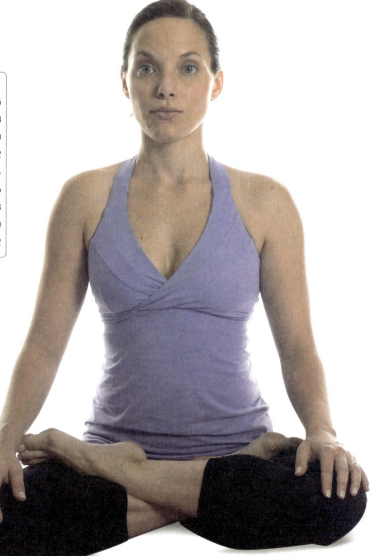

Seated & Seated Twist Poses

Seated postures allow you to practice meditation or work on different breathing exercises (Pranayama). If you have a tight lower back or tight hamstrings, try sitting on a block or blanket to help create length and space in the spine. Seated twists are practiced to help detoxify the body. Each time you twist, you are "massaging" your internal organs and helping to improve your digestion. All too often, the hips tend to do the twisting; instead, keep your hips square and your pelvis level. Imagine wringing out a washcloth as you inhale to lengthen the spine and exhale to twist deeper.

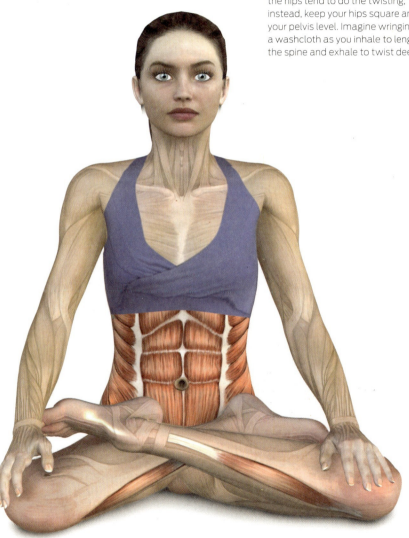

Staff Pose

(Dandasana)

Staff Pose is the Mountain Pose of the seated postures. It forms the basis for many of the other seated poses.

1 Sit up tall, with your legs together and extended in front of you. Firm your thighs into the floor, activating your legs. Flex your feet, drawing your toes back toward your face as you press your heels forward.

2 Find a neutral pelvis, sitting toward the fronts of your sitting bones as your tailbone roots down toward the floor. Position your arms by your sides, with your hands pressed into the floor.

3 Engage your stomach muscles, lifting energy upward—from the base of your tailbone to the crown of your head. Hold for 1 to 5 breaths, or remain in the pose longer if desired.

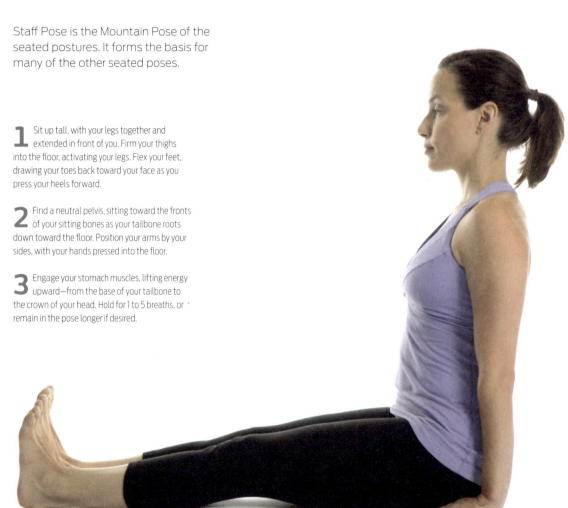

Correct form
- Keep your legs firm and active.
- Draw your shoulder blades together.
- If you find that you lower back is rounding and your pelvis tucks under when your legs are straight, try sitting on a block or blanket.

Avoid
- Letting your legs become soft.
- Sticking your ribs outward.

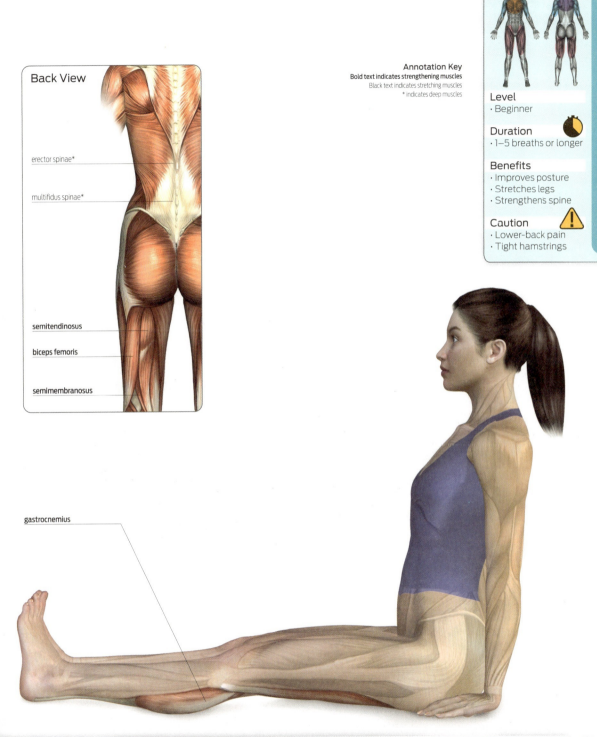

ANATOMY OF FITNESS • YOGA

Easy Pose
(Sukhasana)

If your hamstrings, lower back, or hip flexors are tight then Easy Pose will not be so easy! As you continue to practice yoga you will find the pose becoming more comfortable—and in time, you'll be able to sit and meditate for hours.

2 Place your hands on your thighs with your palms facing either up or down.

3 Close your eyes and draw your focus inward. Lengthen your inhalation and exhalation, aiming for equal length. Try to match the length of your exhale to your inhale. Hold for 1 to 5 breaths, or remain in the pose longer if desired.

1 Sit on the floor, bend your knees, and cross your legs at the shins. Flex your feet to keep your knees in alignment. Feel both sitting bones firmly pressing into the floor and find a neutral pelvis. Lengthen your spine by sitting up straight and opening up across your collarbones.

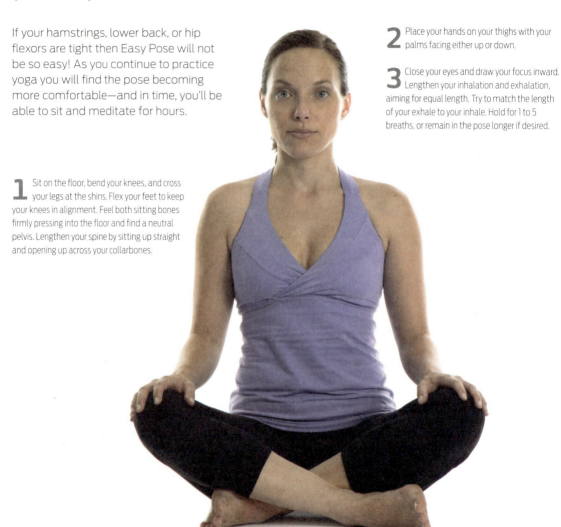

Correct form
- Sit on a block or blanket to elevate your hips above your knees.
- Alternate the crossing of your shins. We all have a dominant side; allow your less dominant side to stretch and find balance in the hips by switching the crossing of your shins.

Avoid
- Letting your knees rise above your hips.
- Rounding your shoulders.

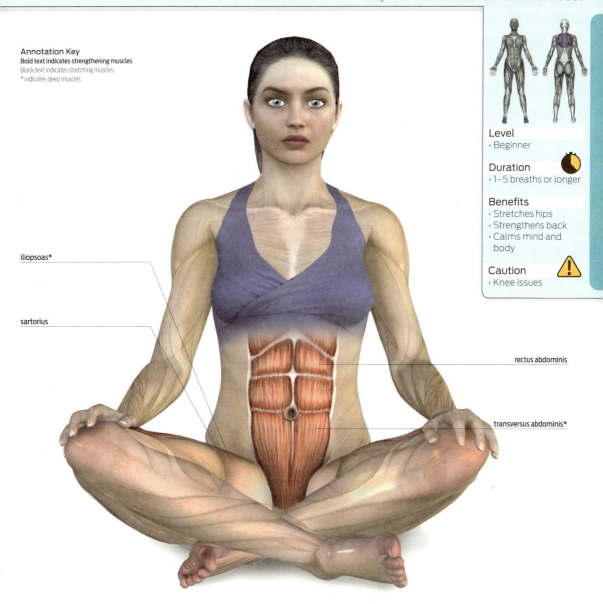
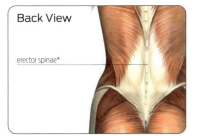

ANATOMY OF FITNESS • YOGA

Hero Pose

(Virasana)

You can sit in Hero to meditate, as an alternative to Full Lotus Pose (pages 134–135) or Easy Pose (pages 128–129).

1 Start in a kneeling position, resting on your knees and shins, with the tops of your feet flat on the floor and toes pointing back.

2 Bring your knees together while moving your feet to slightly wider than hip-width apart. You can use your fingers on the backs of your knees to roll the flesh of your calves down toward your heels.

3 Sit your buttocks down between your heels, keeping your torso upright. Find internal rotation in your thighs, pressing them downward. Lengthen your tailbone down toward your heels as you lift your pubic bone up toward your belly button.

4 Rest your hands on your thighs with the palms facing up in a gesture of receiving and energizing or down for a more grounding and calming effect. Hold for 1 to 5 breaths, or remain in the pose longer if desired.

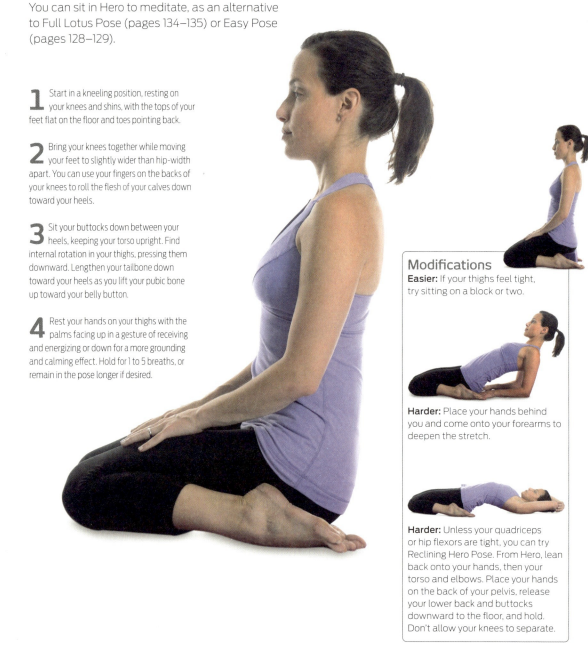

Modifications
Easier: If your thighs feel tight, try sitting on a block or two.

Harder: Place your hands behind you and come onto your forearms to deepen the stretch.

Harder: Unless your quadriceps or hip flexors are tight, you can try Reclining Hero Pose. From Hero, lean back onto your hands, then your torso and elbows. Place your hands on the back of your pelvis, release your lower back and buttocks downward to the floor, and hold. Don't allow your knees to separate.

Hero Pose • **SEATED & SEATED TWIST POSES**

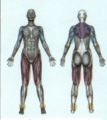

Level
· Beginner

Duration
· 1–5 breaths or longer

Benefits
· Stretches thighs, knees, and ankles

Caution
· Ankle issues
· Knee issues

Annotation Key
Bold text indicates strengthening muscles
Black text indicates stretching muscles
* indicates deep muscles

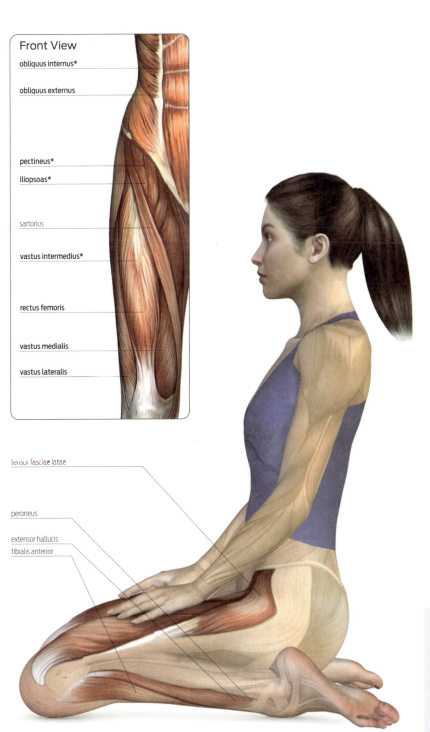

Front View
- obliquus internus*
- obliquus externus
- pectineus*
- iliopsoas*
- sartorius
- vastus intermedius*
- rectus femoris
- vastus medialis
- vastus lateralis
- tensor fasciae latae
- peroneus
- extensor hallucis
- tibialis anterior

Correct form
· Draw your shoulders back and your shoulder blades toward each other.
· If your thighs feel tight, try elevating your hips on blocks.

Avoid
· Sticking your ribs outward.
· Practicing this pose if you experience any knee pain or discomfort with your knees bent.

131

Cow-Face Pose

(Gomukhasana)

It can be difficult to practice all of the components of Cow-Face Pose correctly at the same time. Like so many other yoga poses, this one improves with diligent practice.

1. Begin in Staff Pose (pages 126–127) with your legs extended forward. Bend your left knee and cross your left leg over your right, positioning your legs so that they cross at the inner thighs. Then, bend your right leg so that the thighs are stacked, one on top of the other. Draw your shins and heels slightly forward.

2. Reach your right arm out to the right, parallel to the floor. Turn your hand to face the ceiling, externally rotate the arm, and reach up by your ear. Bend your elbow so that it points toward the ceiling as your fingers point down your spine.

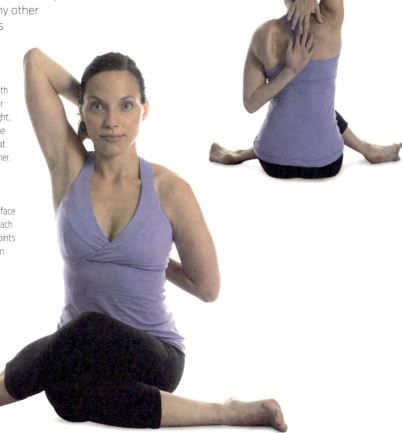

3. Reach your left arm out to the left, parallel to the floor, internally rotating the arm and allowing the hand to face behind you and the thumb to point downward. Bend your arm, pointing your elbow toward the floor, and bring the hand behind your back, palm away from your body and fingers pointing up the spine.

4. Bring your hands toward each other, clasp them together, and hold for 1 to 5 breaths. Repeat on the other side.

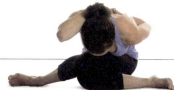

Modifications
Harder: Lengthen your spine, lift your top elbow upward, and lift your chest as you fold forward. Keep your legs in place and your hips facing forward as you hold.

Cow-Face Pose • **SEATED & SEATED TWIST POSES**

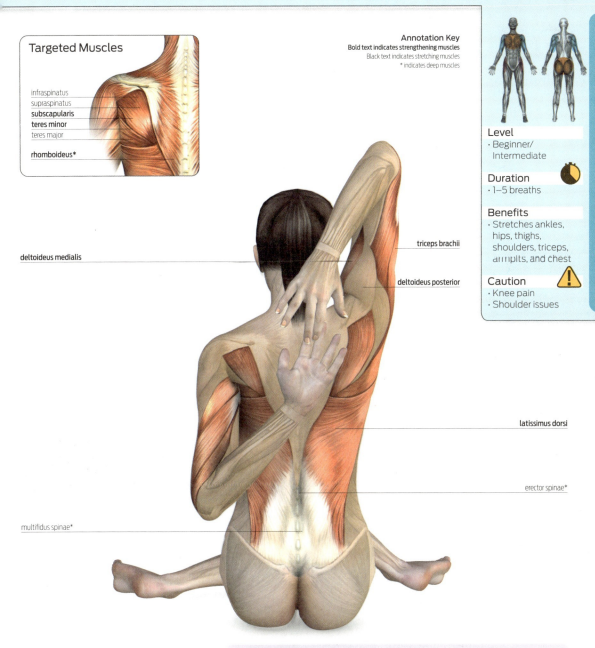

Targeted Muscles

infraspinatus
supraspinatus
subscapularis
teres minor
teres major
rhomboideus*

Annotation Key
Bold text indicates strengthening muscles
Black text indicates stretching muscles
* indicates deep muscles

deltoideus medialis
triceps brachii
deltoideus posterior
latissimus dorsi
erector spinae*
multifidus spinae*

Level
- Beginner/Intermediate

Duration
- 1–5 breaths

Benefits
- Stretches ankles, hips, thighs, shoulders, triceps, armpits, and chest

Caution
- Knee pain
- Shoulder issues

Correct form
- Position your feet so that the right and left are the same distance from your hips.
- If your hips are uneven when you are sitting on the floor, sit on top of a block or a blanket.
- If your hands don't reach each other right away, try using a strap.
- Draw your elbows in opposite directions as you hold the pose.
- Keep your head and gaze forward.

Avoid
- Allowing someone else to push your hands together, as this can strain your shoulder or rotator cuff.

ANATOMY OF FITNESS • YOGA

Full Lotus Pose

(Padmasana)

A highly effective hip opener, Full Lotus Pose is commonly used for meditation. You can build up to the full pose by starting with Half Lotus Pose until you feel comfortable with this advanced position.

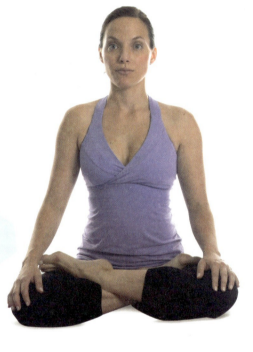

1 Begin in Staff Pose (pages 126–127), and then bend your knees into Easy Pose (pages 128–129). Use your hands to lift your right foot and shin up, drawing the right heel in toward your left hip and resting the foot on your left thigh. If you'd like, you can skip step 2, keeping your legs in this position and proceeding through steps 3 and 4 to complete Half Lotus Pose (Ardha Padmasana).

2 Position your left foot on top of your right thigh so that both feet are resting on the opposite thighs. Hook your ankles as far as possible up your thighs, drawing them toward your hips. Flex your feet; this helps to keep your knees and ankles in alignment.

3 Balance both sitting bones and press them evenly into the floor. Externally rotate your hips, feeling your inner knees opening away from each other. Find a neutral pelvis, drawing your tailbone toward the floor. Draw your stomach in toward your spine.

4 Sit up tall, lengthening from your torso and broadening across your collarbones to lift your sternum. Imagine your chest opening as you allow your arms to draw open. Position your hands either facing up in a gesture of receiving, or facing down in a gesture of grounding. Close your eyes as you hold for at least 5 breaths. Repeat on the other side.

Full Lotus Pose • **SEATED & SEATED TWIST POSES**

Annotation Key
Bold text indicates strengthening muscles
Black text indicates stretching muscles
* indicates deep muscles

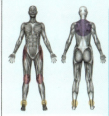

Level
• Advanced

Duration
• 5 breaths or longer

Benefits
• Stretches hips, thighs, knees, ankles, and buttocks
• Stimulates digestion
• Calms mind and body

Caution
• Ankle issues
• Hip issues
• Knee issues

rectus abdominis

obliquus externus

obliquus internus*

transversus abdominis*

tibialis anterior

Correct form
• Keep your back straight; if you have trouble doing so, place a folded blanket beneath your hips to lift them above your knees.
• Switch the crossing of your legs, holding the position for the same duration on both sides.
• Keep your upper body straight and your torso long.

Avoid
• Straining your knees by trying to adopt the pose when you're not yet ready.
• Overextending your outer ankles.
• Leaning or tilting your upper body to one side.

ANATOMY OF FITNESS • YOGA

Full Boat Pose

(Paripurna Navasana)

Full Boat Pose builds incredible core strength and stability. The more you practice it, the more you'll feel your deep stomach muscles and hip flexors working.

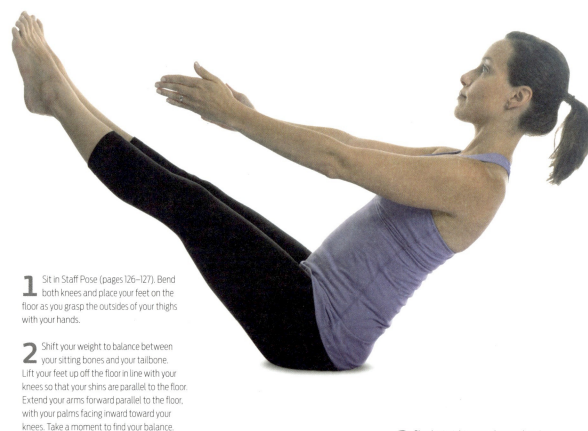

1 Sit in Staff Pose (pages 126–127). Bend both knees and place your feet on the floor as you grasp the outsides of your thighs with your hands.

2 Shift your weight to balance between your sitting bones and your tailbone. Lift your feet up off the floor in line with your knees so that your shins are parallel to the floor. Extend your arms forward parallel to the floor, with your palms facing inward toward your knees. Take a moment to find your balance.

3 Slowly straighten your legs so that they form a 45-degree angle, with your toes lifted very slightly higher than your head.

4 Internally rotate your thighs as you firm your outer hips in to find stability. Squeeze your legs together as if they were a single leg, reaching out through your fingers and toes as you lift your sternum to broaden across your collarbones. Lengthen your spine and engage your stomach muscles as you hold for 1 to 5 breaths.

Modifications

Easier: You can hold the pose after step 2, keeping your legs bent as your feet stay in line with your knees and your shins stay parallel to the floor.

Full Boat Pose • **SEATED & SEATED TWIST POSES**

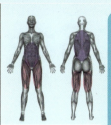

Annotation Key
Bold text indicates strengthening muscles
Black text indicates stretching muscles
* indicates deep muscles

Correct form
• Draw your belly button in toward your spine.
• Maintain the position of your legs, keeping them active and strong.
• Draw your sacrum into your body; this will help to keep your spine long and straight.

Avoid
• Letting your legs drop downward.
• Rounding your lower back.
• Allowing your stomach to bulge outward.

Level
• Beginner/Intermediate

Duration
• 1–5 breaths

Benefits
• Strengthens stomach, back, and hip flexors
• Aids digestion

Caution
• Pregnancy

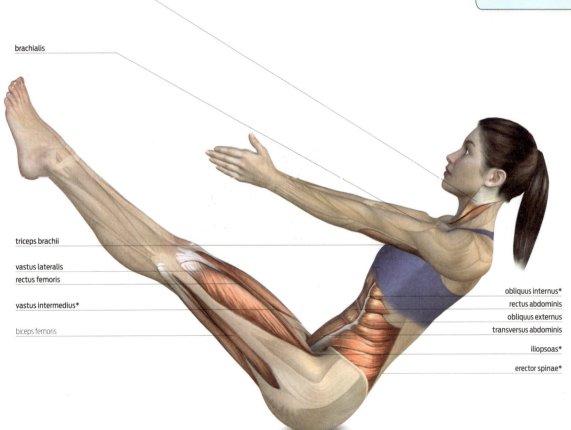

sternocleidomastoideus
brachialis
triceps brachii
vastus lateralis
rectus femoris
vastus intermedius*
biceps femoris
obliquus internus*
rectus abdominis
obliquus externus
transversus abdominis
iliopsoas*
erector spinae*

137

Sage's Pose
(Marichyasana III)

This simple seated twist will both stretch and strengthen your spine.

1 Sit in Staff Pose (pages 126–127), with both legs extended in front of you. Bend your left knee and place the sole of your foot on the floor beside your right knee. Press the right thigh down toward the floor, finding a slight internal rotation, and flex your right foot, grounding down with the heel and drawing the toes back toward your face.

2 Place your left hand on the floor behind your left hip, fingers pointing back. Inhaling, lift your right arm to find length on the right side of your body.

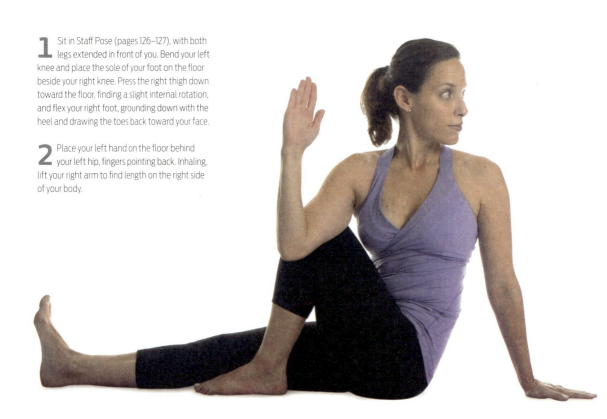

3 Exhaling, twist your upper body to the left and bring your right elbow to the outside of your left knee.

4 Ground down evenly through both sitting bones. Hold for 1 to 5 breaths. Repeat on the other side.

Correct form
- Twist from your spine.
- Keep your bent knee upright.
- Keep your extended knee straight and activated.
- Press down into the floor with the foot of your bent knee.

Avoid
- Twisting your neck into an uncomfortable position.
- Allowing your extended leg to turn out.

Sage's Pose • **SEATED & SEATED TWIST POSES**

Level
• Beginner

Duration
• 1–5 breaths

Benefits
• Aids digestion
• Stretches and strengthens spine
• Stretches shoulders

Caution
• Back issues

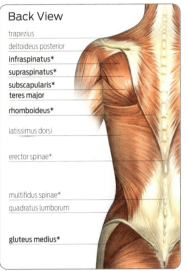

Back View
- trapezius
- deltoideus posterior
- **infraspinatus***
- **supraspinatus***
- **subscapularis***
- teres major
- **rhomboideus***
- latissimus dorsi
- erector spinae*
- multifidus spinae*
- quadratus lumborum
- **gluteus medius***

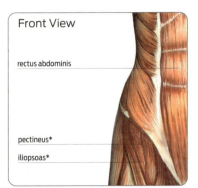

Front View
- rectus abdominis
- pectineus*
- iliopsoas*

Annotation Key
Bold text indicates strengthening muscles
Black text indicates stretching muscles
* indicates deep muscles

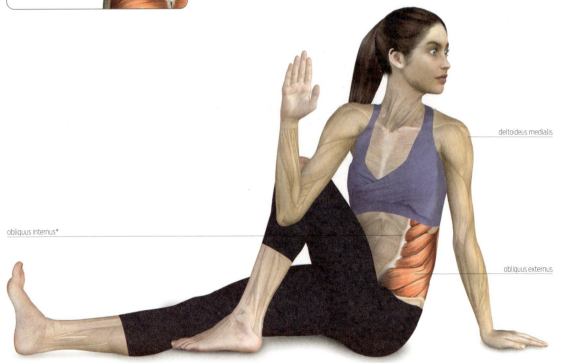

- obliquus internus*
- deltoideus medialis
- obliquus externus

ANATOMY OF FITNESS • YOGA

Half Lord of the Fishes Pose

(Ardha Matsyendrasana)

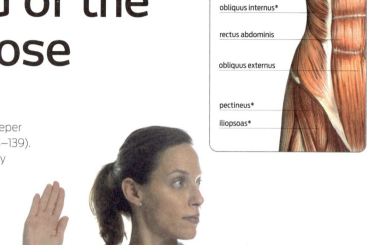

Half Lord of the Fishes Pose is a deeper variation of Sage's Pose (pages 138–139). This seated spinal twist will not only stretch the spine, but it will also open your hips and shoulders.

1 Sit in Staff Pose (pages 126–127), with both legs extended in front of you. Bend your left knee, and place your left foot on the outside of your right leg, resting flat on the floor. Your left knee should point straight up toward the ceiling.

2 Shift your weight slightly to the left as you bend your right leg inward and bring the heel close to your left hip.

3 Place your left hand on the floor behind your left hip, fingers pointing back. Inhaling, lift your right arm to find length on the right side of your body.

4 Exhaling, twist your upper body to the left and bring your right elbow to the outside of your left knee. Ground down evenly through both sitting bones.

5 To deepen the twist, find resistance between your arm and your bent leg. If desired, turn your gaze over your left shoulder, and raise your right hand, palm turned away from the body. Hold for 1 to 5 breaths. Repeat on the other side.

Correct form
- Sit up tall and lengthen your spine as you twist.
- Distribute your weight evenly between both sitting bones; if you find that your hips are uneven, try sitting on top of a block or a blanket.
- Broaden across your collarbones.
- Draw your shoulder blades together.
- Ground down through your tailbone.

Avoid
- Twisting your neck into an uncomfortable position.

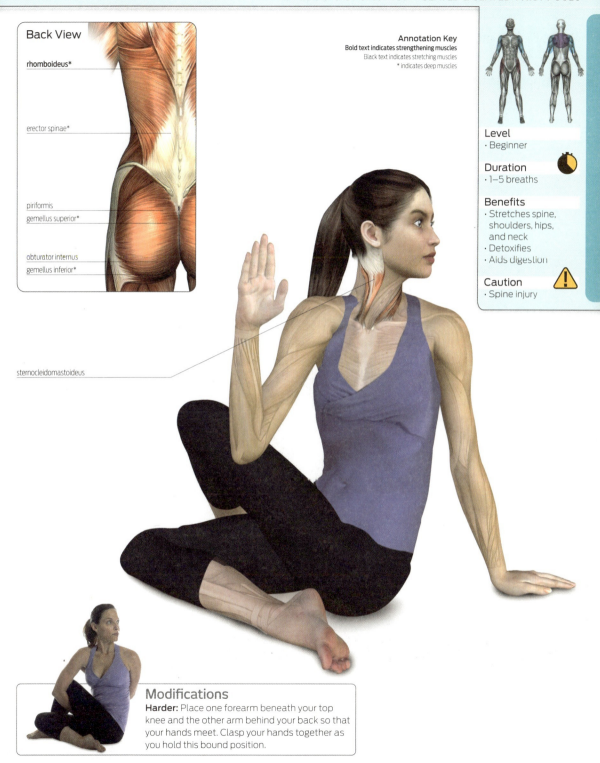

Monkey Pose

(Hanumanasana)

Monkey Pose is deeply challenging. It requires time, patience, and practice as you build up to performing the full split.

1 Kneel on the floor, with your back straight and your arms at your sides. Step your right foot forward to come into Low Lunge (pages 52–53), and place your fingertips on the floor on either side of your foot.

2 Extend your right leg forward, flexing the foot so that your heel is on the floor and your toes point toward you. Feel free to pause in this position, taking several breaths as you stretch your hamstrings.

3 Slide your right heel forward, keeping your right leg straight. Continue to slide forward until your left leg is also straight. Keep your hips square by thinking of drawing your right hip crease back and your left hip forward.

4 Inhale your arms straight above your head and keep them shoulder-width apart, fingers reaching toward the ceiling. Hold for 1 to 5 breaths. Repeat on the other side.

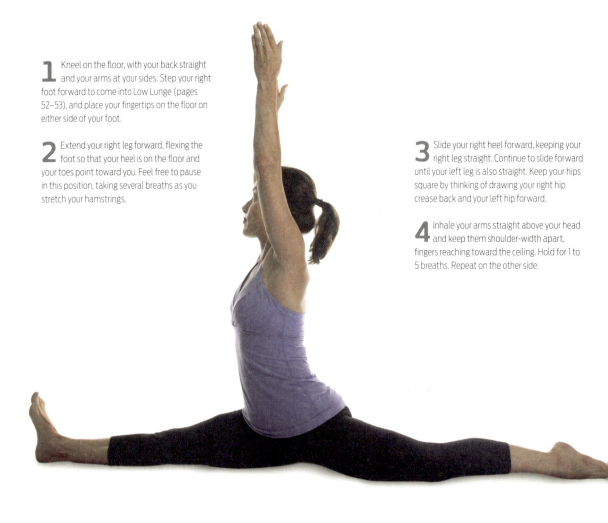

Monkey Pose • **SEATED & SEATED TWIST POSES**

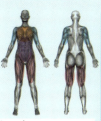

Level
· Intermediate/ Advanced

Duration
· 1–5 breaths

Benefits
· Stretches hamstrings, groin, thighs, and hips

Caution
· Groin issues
· Hamstring issues

Correct form
· Ease your way into the split.
· As you descend, push into the floor with your front heel and the top of your back foot.

Avoid
· Allowing the hip of your back leg to turn outward.
· Forcing yourself into the full pose when you are not yet ready.

Annotation Key
Bold text indicates strengthening muscles
Black text indicates stretching muscles
* indicates deep muscles

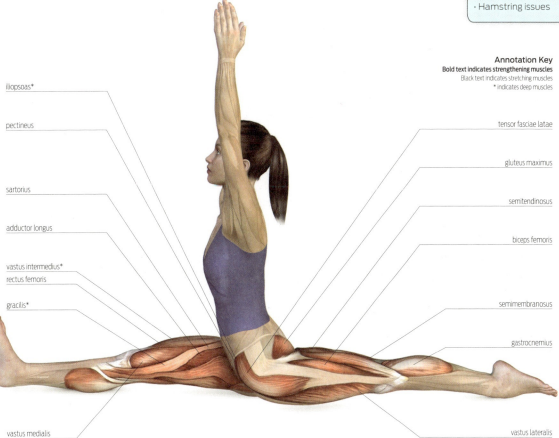

iliopsoas*
pectineus
sartorius
adductor longus
vastus intermedius*
rectus femoris
gracilis*
vastus medialis

tensor fasciae latae
gluteus maximus
semitendinosus
biceps femoris
semimembranosus
gastrocnemius
vastus lateralis

ANATOMY OF FITNESS • YOGA

Contents

Child's Pose	146
Extended Puppy Pose	148
Bound Angle Pose	150
Fire Log Pose	152
Head-to-Knee Forward Bend	154
Revolved Head-to-Knee Pose	156
Seated Forward Bend	158
Wide-Angle Seated Forward Bend	160

SEATED FORWARD BENDS

Seated Forward Bends

Cooling and calming, seated forward bends are often part of yoga classes' closing sequences. They require you to dig within yourself, as they are introspective and therapeutic. Lengthen your exhalations as you fold deeper into your forward bends, and, if you feel comfortable, try closing your eyes. Seated forward bends are thought to improve digestion. They can also be helpful for improving mild depression, headaches, anxiety, and stress.

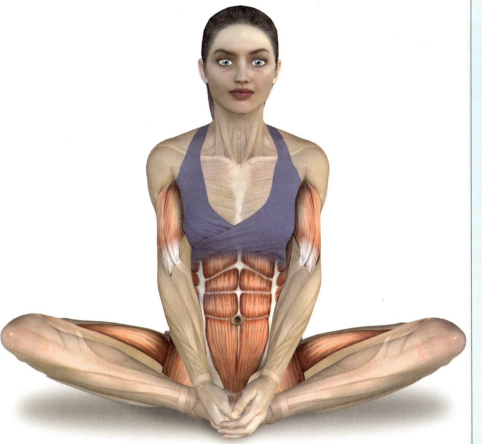

ANATOMY OF FITNESS • YOGA

Child's Pose

(Balasana)

Very relaxing and restorative, Child's Pose is a perfect resting position which you can assume at any point during your practice.

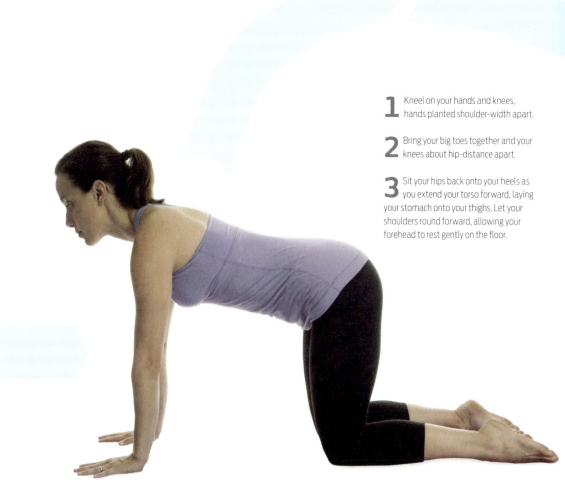

1 Kneel on your hands and knees, hands planted shoulder-width apart.

2 Bring your big toes together and your knees about hip-distance apart.

3 Sit your hips back onto your heels as you extend your torso forward, laying your stomach onto your thighs. Let your shoulders round forward, allowing your forehead to rest gently on the floor.

Correct form
- Relax any tension you may be holding in your jaw and face muscles.
- Open up between your shoulder blades as you breathe.

Avoid
- Bringing your knees too far apart.

Child's Pose • **SEATED FORWARD BENDS**

4 Bring your arms by your sides with the palms of your hands facing upward. Breathe into the back of your body. Hold for 5 to 10 breaths.

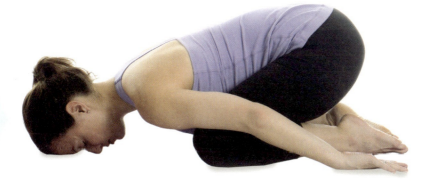

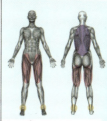

Level
• Beginner

Duration
• 5–10 breaths

Benefits
• Reduces stress and anxiety
• Aids digestion
• Relieves back pain
• Stretches ankles, back, and hips

Caution
• Knee issues

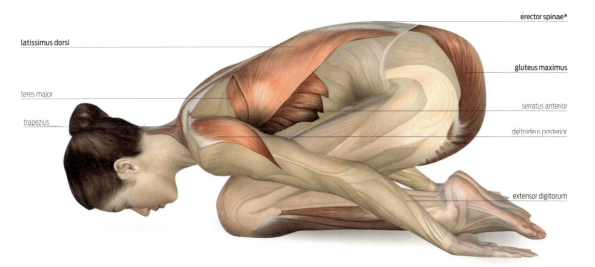

erector spinae*
gluteus maximus
serratus anterior
deltoideus posterior
extensor digitorum

latissimus dorsi
teres major
trapezius

Annotation Key
Bold text indicates strengthening muscles
Black text indicates stretching muscles
* indicates deep muscles

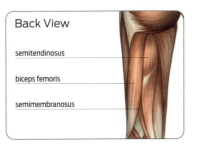

Back View
semitendinosus
biceps femoris
semimembranosus

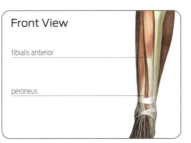

Front View
tibialis anterior
peroneus

147

Extended Puppy Pose

(Uttana Shishosana)

Extended Puppy Pose is a resting posture, combining the shoulder and arm stretch of Downward-Facing Dog with the relaxing quality of Child's Pose.

1 Begin on your hands and knees with your hands beneath your shoulders and your knees directly below your hips.

2 Keep your knees in place as you walk your hands forward and stretch your arms straight. Externally rotate your outer upper arms toward your ears. Keep your arms active.

3 Adopt a Downward-Facing Dog (pages 116–117) position in your upper body, with your hands shoulder width apart, fingers widely spread, and hands pressed down to lengthen your spine. Resist your forearms away from the floor to keep your elbows lifted.

4 Bring your belly in to support your lower back as you stretch.

5 Let your forehead rest toward the floor and allow your neck to soften. Close your eyes and hold for 1 to 5 breaths.

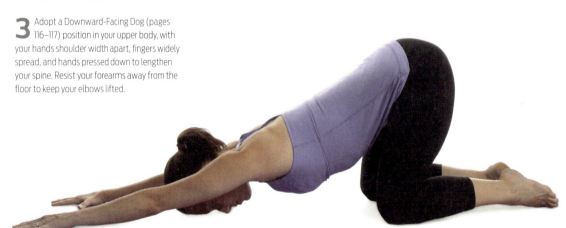

Correct form
· Keep your neck and shoulders soft.

Avoid
· Letting your ribs jut forward.
· Sinking into your lower back.

Extended Puppy Pose • **SEATED FORWARD BENDS**

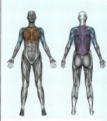

Annotation Key
Bold text indicates strengthening muscles
Black text indicates stretching muscles
* indicates deep muscles

Level
- Beginner

Duration
- 1–5 breaths

Benefits
- Lengthens spine
- Stretches shoulders
- Relaxes mind and body

Caution
- Knee issues
- Lower-back issues

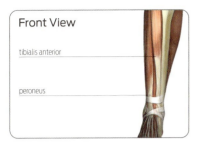

Front View
tibialis anterior
peroneus

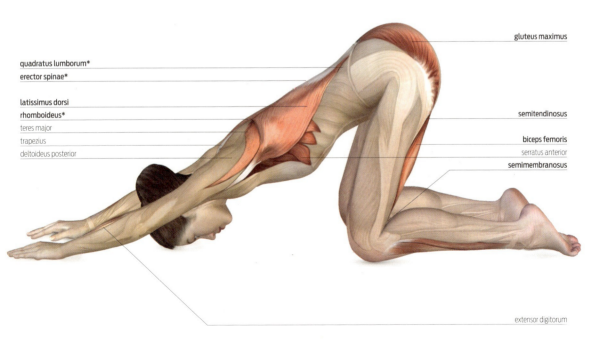

quadratus lumborum*
erector spinae*
latissimus dorsi
rhomboideus*
teres major
trapezius
deltoideus posterior

gluteus maximus
semitendinosus
biceps femoris
serratus anterior
semimembranosus
extensor digitorum

149

ANATOMY OF FITNESS • YOGA

Bound Angle Pose
(Baddha Konasana)

Beneficial for all levels, Bound Angle Pose is a great hip opener. To execute this pose properly, aim your navel—not your head—toward your feet.

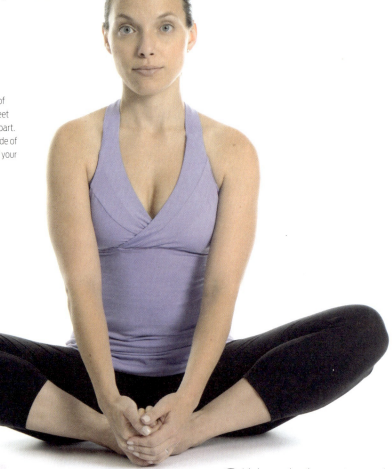

1 Sit in Staff Pose (pages 126–127).

2 Bend both knees and bring the soles of your feet together as you draw your feet in toward your pelvis, keeping your knees apart. Hold your ankles and press the small-toe side of both feet together, "opening" the insides of your feet as if you were opening a book.

3 Inhale as you lengthen your sternum and open your collarbones. Exhale and fold forward if desired, leading with your heart. Hold for 5 to 20 breaths.

Correct form
- Create a straight line from your sitting bones to your shoulders: lift upward from your spine, and press your chest and shoulders open.
- To make the pose feel more restorative, try resting your forehead on a block.

Avoid
- Rounding your upper back to fold forward.
- Forcing your knees down.

Bound Angle Pose • **SEATED FORWARD BENDS**

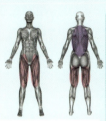

Level
• Beginner

Duration
• 5–20 breaths

Benefits
• Stretches inner and outer thighs, groin, and spine
• Calms mind

Caution
• Groin issues

Front View

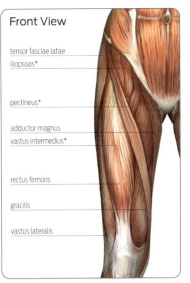

- tensor fasciae latae
- iliopsoas*
- pectineus*
- adductor magnus
- vastus intermedius*
- rectus femoris
- gracilis
- vastus lateralis

Back View

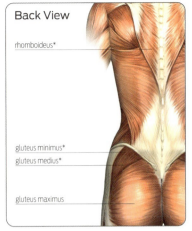

- rhomboideus*
- gluteus minimus*
- gluteus medius*
- gluteus maximus

Annotation Key
Bold text indicates strengthening muscles
Black text indicates stretching muscles
* indicates deep muscles

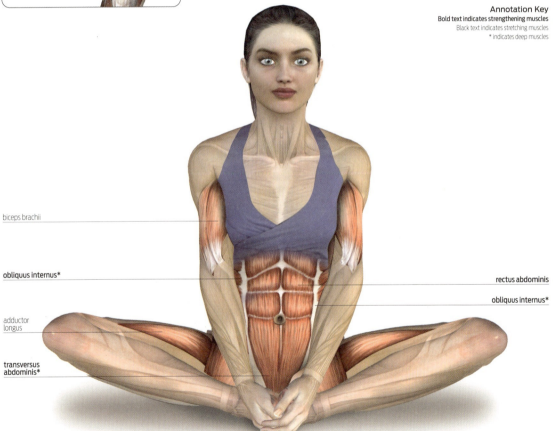

- biceps brachii
- obliquus internus*
- adductor longus
- transversus abdominis*
- rectus abdominis
- obliquus internus*

151

ANATOMY OF FITNESS • YOGA

Fire Log Pose
(Agnistambhasana)

Fire Log Pose is a very deep hip opener and buttocks stretch. Practice this pose toward the end of your yoga session once you have built heat and loosened your hips joints.

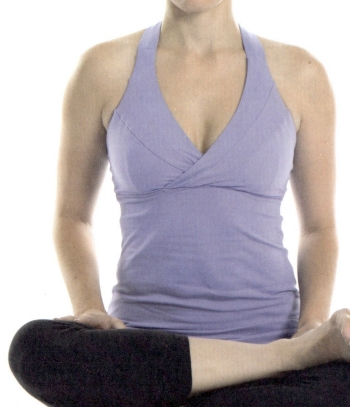

1 Sit in Staff Pose (pages 126–127).

2 Bend your right knee and place your right ankle over your straight left knee. Bend your left leg under and place your left ankle beneath your right knee, stacking ankle over knee so that your shins are parallel to each other. Flex both feet and press out through your heels to keep both knees in alignment.

3 You may find that this is enough of a hip stretch for you, especially if your right knee is lifting high up off of your left ankle. You can stay here and feel your hips opening—or, to deepen the stretch, inhale and lengthen your torso, then exhale and fold forward from your hips. Hold for 5 to 10 breaths.

Correct form
- Keep your spine long, even as you fold forward.
- Roll the flesh of your buttocks out from under you before folding forward.

Avoid
- Letting your feet and ankles cave inward.
- Rounding your shoulders or upper back as you fold forward.

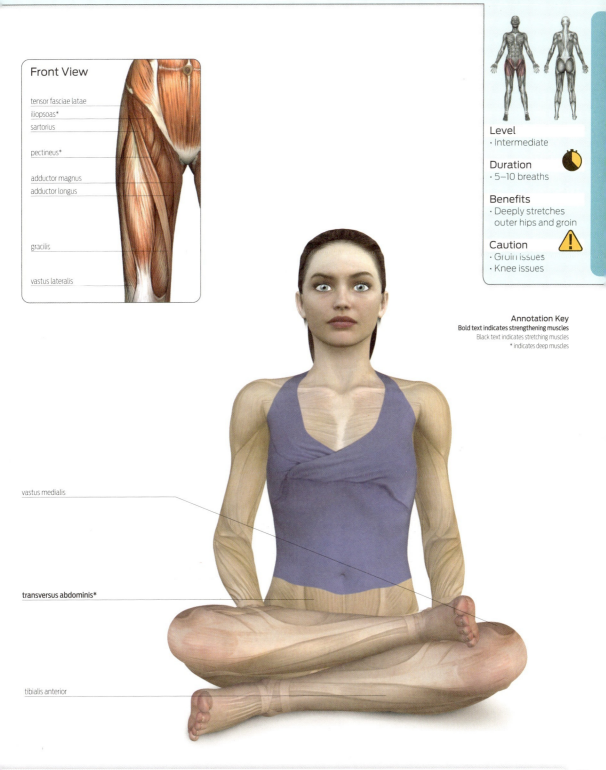

ANATOMY OF FITNESS • YOGA

Head-to-Knee Forward Bend

(Janu Sirsasana)

Head-to-Knee Forward Bend offers a slight twist, as well as an excellent stretch for your hamstrings, hips, and the back of your body.

1 Sit up tall in Staff Pose (pages 126–127). Bend your left leg out to the left, externally rotating the hip. Place the sole of your left foot on the inner thigh of your right leg.

2 Activate your extended right leg by firming your thigh down toward the floor. Slightly internally rotate your thigh to keep the leg in a neutral position.

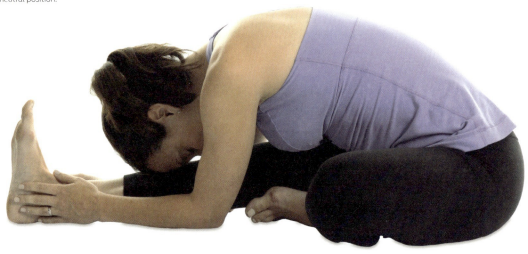

3 Lengthen your spine, drawing energy down from your tailbone as you reach energy up through the crown of your head. Inhale your arms above your head so that they are parallel to each other.

4 Lengthen your torso, turning it slightly to the right as you exhale and hinge forward with a flat back, reaching your arms toward your right foot. Hold for 5 breaths. Repeat on the other side.

Head-to-Knee Forward Bend • **SEATED FORWARD BENDS**

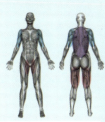

Correct form
- Fold more from your hips than from your waist. To help you do this, allow your pelvis to tilt back and your sacrum to move toward your lower back as you bend forward.
- Let your head drop down.
- Soften your shoulders, releasing tension.

Avoid
- Rounding your spine forward. It isn't necessary to touch your toes; if you notice that your spine rounds when you bend forward, try bringing your hands onto your shins or using a strap.

Level
- Beginner

Duration
- 5 breaths

Benefits
- Stretches spine, shoulders, groin, hips, and hamstrings
- Calms mind

Caution
- Knee issues

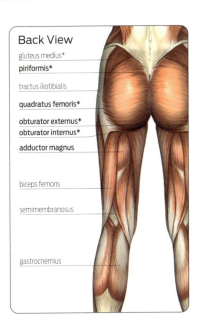

Back View
- gluteus medius*
- **piriformis***
- tractus iliotibialis
- **quadratus femoris***
- **obturator externus***
- **obturator internus***
- **adductor magnus**
- biceps femoris
- semimembranosus
- gastrocnemius

Annotation Key
Bold text indicates strengthening muscles
Black text indicates stretching muscles
* indicates deep muscles

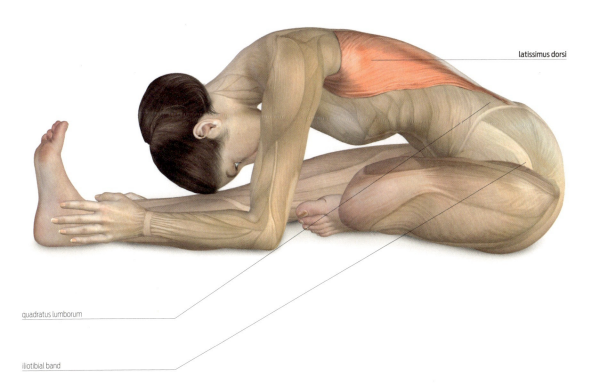

latissimus dorsi

quadratus lumborum

iliotibial band

155

Revolved Head-to-Knee Pose

(Parivrtta Janu Sirsasana)

As you practice Revolved Head-to-Knee Pose, the counter-pose to Head-to-Knee Forward Bend, you will feel a deep stretch along the side of your body.

1 Sit up tall in Staff Pose (pages 126–127). Bend your left leg out to the left, externally rotating the hip. Place the sole of your left foot on the inner thigh of your right leg.

2 Bring your right foot slightly to the right, externally rotate your hip, and open your left leg out to the left to widen the foundation.

3 Place your right forearm on the inside of your right shin. Grasp the inside of your right foot.

4 Reach your left arm toward the ceiling and outwardly rotate the arm, bringing it over your left ear. Bend to the right, reaching for the outside of your right foot with your left hand.

5 Nestle your right shoulder toward the inside of your right leg, slightly bend both elbows away from each other, and lean back. Use this resistance to twist your right ribs and torso toward the ceiling. Hold for 5 breaths. Repeat on the other side.

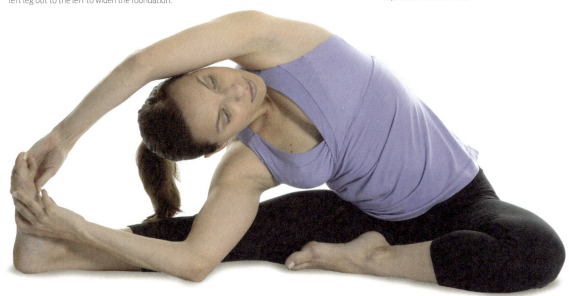

Correct form
· Activate your extended leg, pressing the thigh into the floor.

Avoid
· Rounding or hunching your shoulders.

Revolved Head-to-Knee Pose • **SEATED FORWARD BENDS**

Back View

trapezius
infraspinatus

rhomboideus
latissimus dorsi

erector spinae*

gluteus medius*

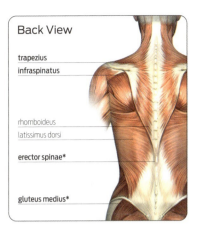

Annotation Key
Bold text indicates strengthening muscles
Black text indicates stretching muscles
* indicates deep muscles

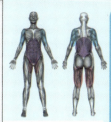

Level
• Beginner

Duration
• 5 breaths

Benefits
• Stretches shoulders, hamstrings, and spine

Caution
• Knee issues
• Lower-back issues

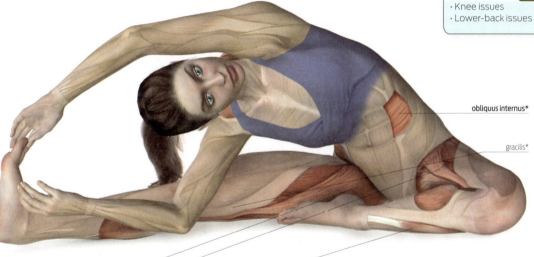

obliquus internus*
gracilis*

adductor magnus
adductor longus

tibialis anterior

Back View

semitendinosus
biceps femoris
semimembranosus
gastrocnemius
soleus

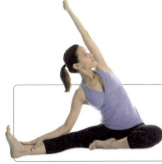

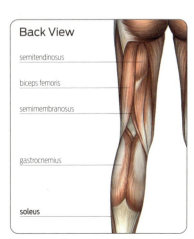

Modifications
Easier: Instead of leaning all the way to the side, place one hand on your shin and extend the other arm over your ear as you bend slightly to the side.

Seated Forward Bend
(Paschimottanasana)

Seated Forward Bend is an introspective posture. With its gesture of surrender, it helps to reduce stress and calm the mind.

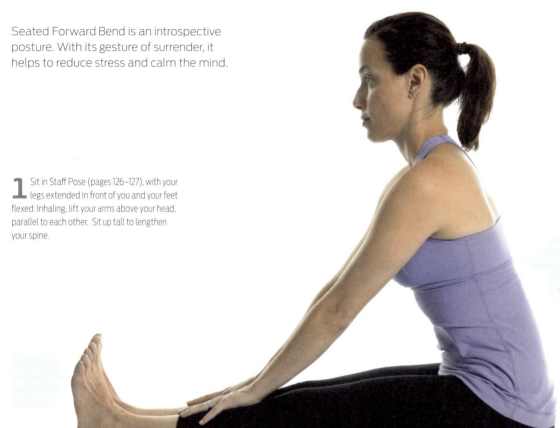

1 Sit in Staff Pose (pages 126–127), with your legs extended in front of you and your feet flexed. Inhaling, lift your arms above your head, parallel to each other. Sit up tall to lengthen your spine.

Correct form
- Keep your feet flexed.
- Try sitting on a blanket if desired.
- To help you fold deeper, think of having a slight arch in your lower back as you root your thighs into the floor.
- Close your eyes if you feel comfortable doing so.
- Try to lengthen your exhalations so that they are longer than your inhalations.

Avoid
- Letting your big toes move farther toward you than the other toes; as you flex, your feet should be straight, as if you were standing on the ground.

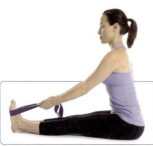

Modifications
Easier: Try placing a strap around the balls of your feet instead of reaching all the way to your feet if your hamstrings and/or lower back feel tight.

Seated Forward Bend • **SEATED FORWARD BENDS**

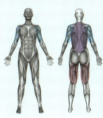

2 Exhaling, fold forward. Grasp the outside of your right foot with your right hand, and the outside of your left foot with your left hand.

3 Hinge at your hips, trying to bring your belly toward your thighs. Allow your head to release downward and hold for 5 to 10 breaths.

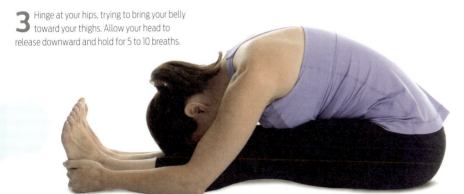

Level
• Beginner

Duration
• 5–10 breaths

Benefits
• Stretches spine, shoulders, and hamstrings
• Calms mind and body

Caution
• Hamstring issues
• Lower-back issues

Annotation Key
Bold text indicates strengthening muscles
Black text indicates stretching muscles
* indicates deep muscles

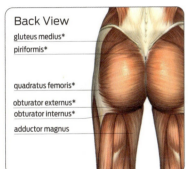

Back View
gluteus medius*
piriformis*
quadratus femoris*
obturator externus*
obturator internus*
adductor magnus

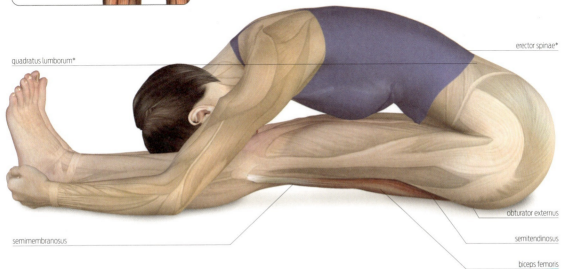

quadratus lumborum*
erector spinae*
obturator externus
semitendinosus
biceps femoris
semimembranosus

159

Wide-Angle Seated Forward Bend

(Upavistha Konasana)

Concentrate on elongating your spine and opening your hips as you practice Wide-Angle Seated Forward Bend—a pose that will challenge your flexibility.

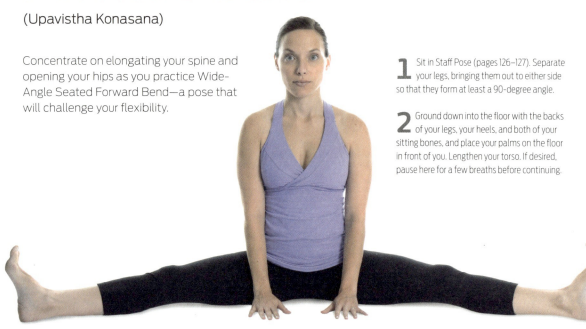

1 Sit in Staff Pose (pages 126–127). Separate your legs, bringing them out to either side so that they form at least a 90-degree angle.

2 Ground down into the floor with the backs of your legs, your heels, and both of your sitting bones, and place your palms on the floor in front of you. Lengthen your torso. If desired, pause here for a few breaths before continuing.

3 Inhaling, lengthen your spine. Exhaling, lengthen your sternum and fold forward, lifting out of your lower back and activating your abdominal muscles. Hold for 5 to 10 breaths.

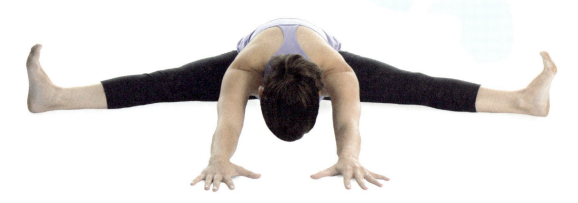

Wide-Angle Seated Forward Bend • SEATED FORWARD BENDS

Correct form
- Keep your toes and kneecaps pointed toward the ceiling.
- If you feel tightness in your hamstrings or lower back, try sitting on top of a blanket or a block.

Avoid
- Forcing your torso to the floor.

Back View

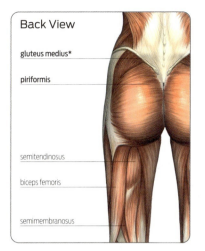

- gluteus medius*
- piriformis
- semitendinosus
- biceps femoris
- semimembranosus

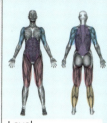

Level
- Beginner

Duration
- 5–10 breaths

Benefits
- Stretches and releases tension in groin and inner and outer thighs
- Strengthens spine

Caution
- Hamstring issues
- Lower-back issues
- Sciatic problems

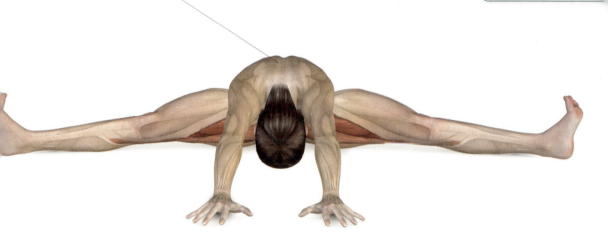

erector spinae*

Front View

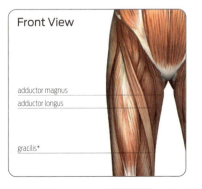

- adductor magnus
- adductor longus
- gracilis*

Annotation Key
Bold text indicates strengthening muscles
Black text indicates stretching muscles
* indicates deep muscles

ANATOMY OF FITNESS • YOGA

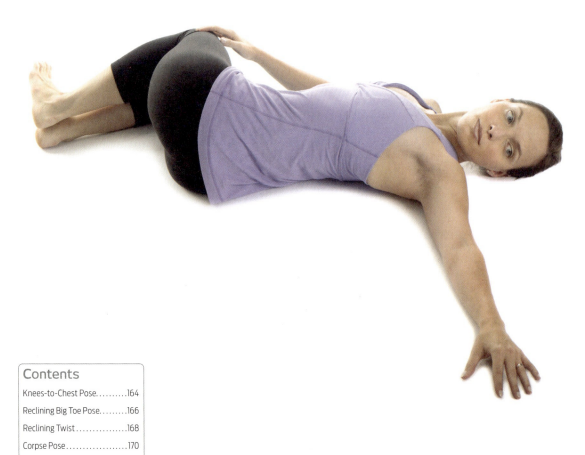

Contents

Knees-to-Chest Pose	164
Reclining Big Toe Pose	166
Reclining Twist	168
Corpse Pose	170

RECLINING POSES

Reclining poses relax and rejuvenate the body and mind, helping you to cool down at the end of the yoga practice. They help to calm the nervous system and relieve tension in the body, giving your muscles a chance to feel the delicious effects of the postures you have just performed. Allow yourself ample time to stay in each reclining pose.

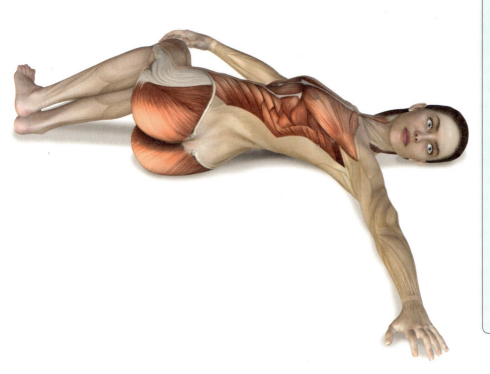

Knees-to-Chest Pose

(Apanasana)

Knees-to-Chest Pose is a relaxing pose that can help to alleviate lower-back pain.

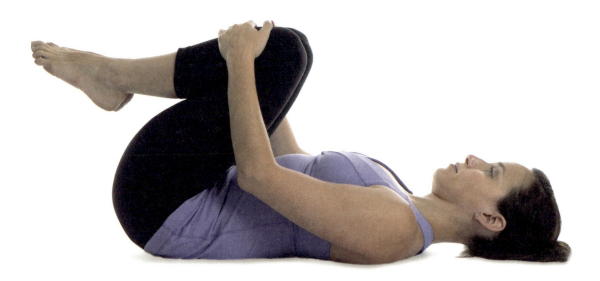

1 Lie on your back. On an exhalation, bend both knees into your chest. Grasp your shins.

2 Draw your shoulders back and hug your knees closer into your chest. Lengthen your tailbone, elongating your spine. Hold for 1 to 5 breaths, gently pulling your knees closer to your chest with each exhalation.

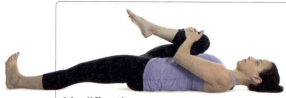

Modifications
Easier: Instead of bringing both knees to your chest, bring just one knee into your chest at a time.

Knees-to-Chest Pose • **RECLINING POSES**

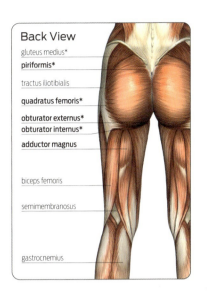

Back View
- gluteus medius*
- **piriformis***
- tractus iliotibialis
- **quadratus femoris***
- **obturator externus***
- **obturator internus***
- **adductor magnus**
- biceps femoris
- semimembranosus
- gastrocnemius

Correct form
- Draw your stomach inward.
- Press down into the floor with your back and shoulders.

Avoid
- Straining your neck; if you have difficulty placing your head on the floor, try resting it on a blanket.

Annotation Key
Bold text indicates strengthening muscles
Black text indicates stretching muscles
* indicates deep muscles

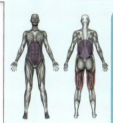

Level
- Beginner

Duration
- 1–5 breaths

Benefits
- Aids digestion
- Helps to alleviate lower-back pain

Caution
- Knee issues
- Pregnancy

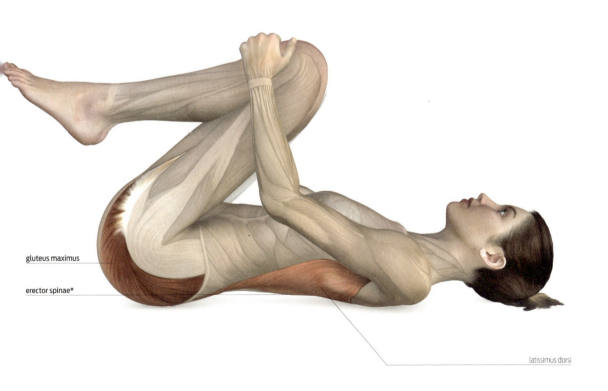

- gluteus maximus
- erector spinae*
- latissimus dorsi

165

Reclining Big Toe Pose
(Supta Padangusthasana)

Very restorative, Reclining Big Toe Pose will improve your flexibility. It is great preparation for Extended Hand-to-Big-Toe Pose (pages 62–63).

1 Lie on your back. Straighten your right leg up toward the ceiling so that the right heel is lined up with the right hip. If possible, continue to extend the leg over the top of your body.

2 With your right hand, grasp your big toe in yogic toe lock with your first two fingers wrapped around the inside of your big toe and your thumb wrapped around the outside of the toe. If desired, bring the leg out to the right to get a deeper stretch in your hip or inner thigh, or cross the leg to the left to stretch your outer hip and IT band.

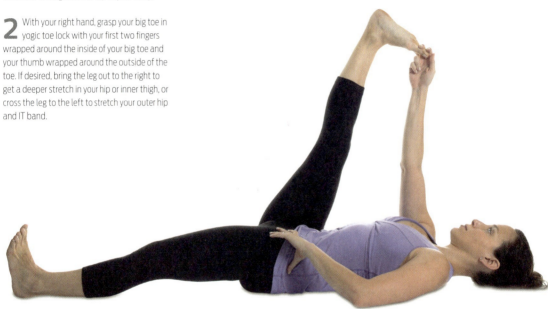

3 Find a slight internal rotation in your right leg. Press your left thigh into the floor as you flex the foot to keep the leg active. Hold for 5 to 10 breaths, gently drawing your right leg toward you to deepen the stretch. Repeat on the other side.

Correct form
- Straighten your lifted leg completely, even if this causes the leg to move away from your head.
- Keep both hips on the floor throughout the exercise.

Avoid
- Allowing the hip on the side of your lifted leg to lift upward.

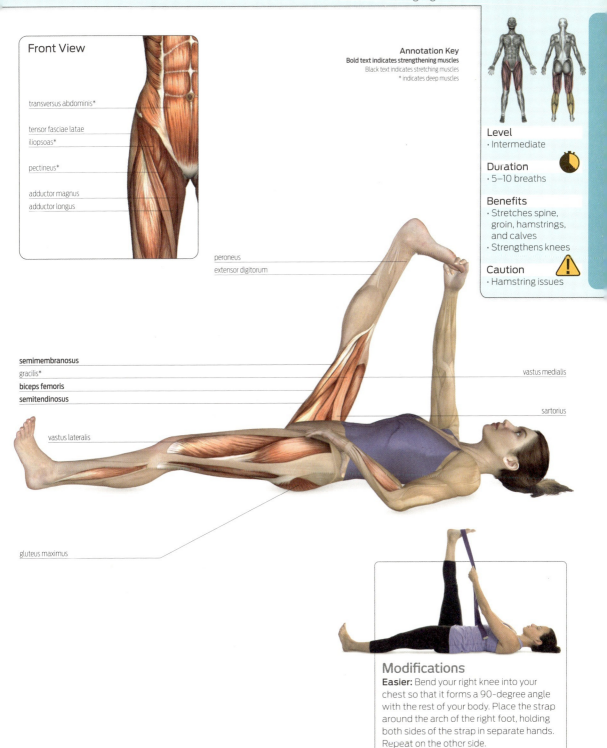

ANATOMY OF FITNESS • YOGA

Reclining Twist
(Jathara Parivrrti)

Reclining Twist can be performed at any level. It is very relaxing, so you can practice it with your eyes closed before moving into Corpse Pose (pages 170–171).

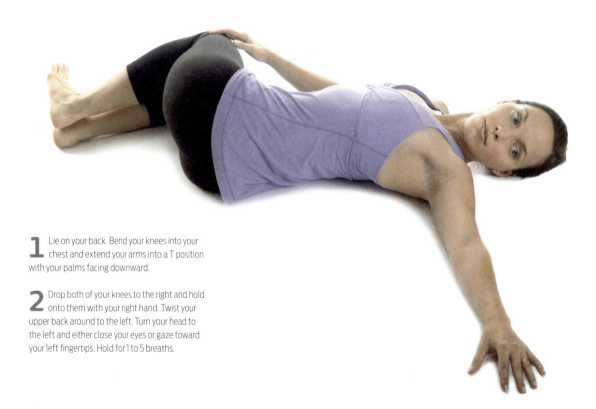

1 Lie on your back. Bend your knees into your chest and extend your arms into a T position with your palms facing downward.

2 Drop both of your knees to the right and hold onto them with your right hand. Twist your upper back around to the left. Turn your head to the left and either close your eyes or gaze toward your left fingertips. Hold for 1 to 5 breaths.

3 Return your knees to center, and then repeat the entire twist in the opposite direction.

Correct form
- Relax into the twist.
- Stack your legs one on top of the other so that the knees, shins, and ankles line up.
- For a deeper twist, lift both shoulders a couple of inches off the floor and then place them back down.

Avoid
- Raising your arms too high if you have shoulder pain.

Reclining Twist • **RECLINING POSES**

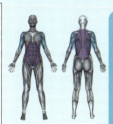

Level
• Beginner

Duration
• 1–5 breaths

Benefits
• Stretches spine
• Aids digestion

Caution
• Lower back issues

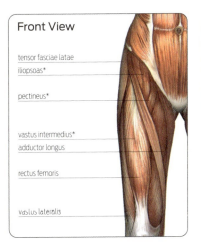

Front View

tensor fasciae latae
iliopsoas*

pectineus*

vastus intermedius*
adductor longus

rectus femoris

vastus lateralis

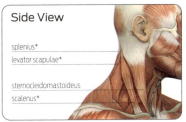

Side View

splenius*
levator scapulae*

sternocleidomastoideus
scalenus*

Annotation Key
Bold text indicates strengthening muscles
Black text indicates stretching muscles
* indicates deep muscles

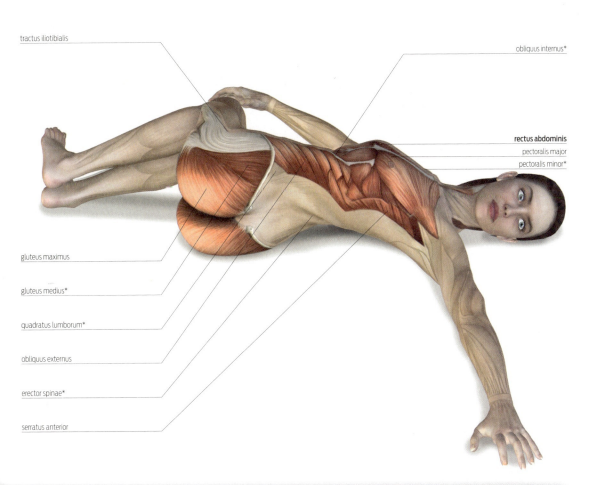

tractus iliotibialis

gluteus maximus

gluteus medius*

quadratus lumborum*

obliquus externus

erector spinae*

serratus anterior

obliquus internus*

rectus abdominis
pectoralis major
pectoralis minor*

169

Corpse Pose
(Savasana)

Corpse Pose, commonly called Savasana, may look easy, but this pose can be highly challenging. Relaxing all your muscles requires total "surrender" and quieting of the body and mind.

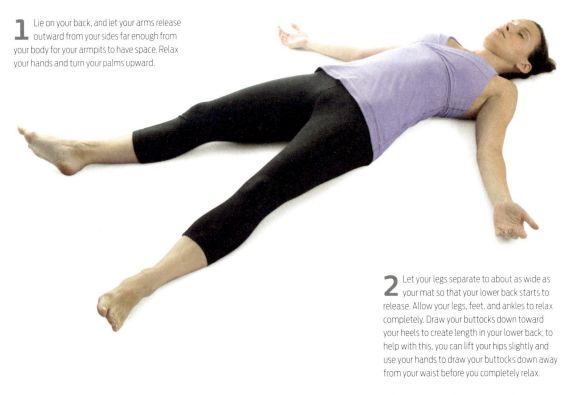

1 Lie on your back, and let your arms release outward from your sides far enough from your body for your armpits to have space. Relax your hands and turn your palms upward.

2 Let your legs separate to about as wide as your mat so that your lower back starts to release. Allow your legs, feet, and ankles to relax completely. Draw your buttocks down toward your heels to create length in your lower back; to help with this, you can lift your hips slightly and use your hands to draw your buttocks down away from your waist before you completely relax.

3 Let your eyes, jaw, tongue, and throat soften. Release any controlled breath, and begin to breathe quietly. Remain here for 3 to 10 minutes, or even longer if desired, before transitioning out of the pose.

Correct form
- Place a rolled-up blanket underneath your knees if you feel any lower-back discomfort.
- Make sure that your body isn't touching anything near your mat, such as your block, strap, or water bottle.

Avoid
- Keeping your eyes open and letting them wander around the room.
- Positioning your body asymmetrically.

Corpse Pose • **RECLINING POSES**

Transitioning Out of Corpse Pose
To transition out of the pose, inhale and exhale deeply and then start to wiggle your fingers and toes, making small movements to bring awareness back to the rest of the body. Hug both knees into your chest, and then gently roll over onto your right side, taking pressure away from the heart. Pause there for a moment in a fetal position. Slowly press yourself up to sit in Easy Pose (pages 128–129), keeping your eyes closed. Stay there for several breaths (or minutes) before opening your eyes.

If you are pregnant, do not lie on your back; instead, lie on your left side or elevate your spine using a block or other booster and as you transition out of the pose, lie in a fetal position on the left side of the body to avoid compromising blood flow to your uterus.

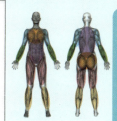

Level
- All levels

Duration
- 3–10 minutes or longer

Benefits
- Encourages deep relaxation
- Calms mind and body
- Decreases depression
- Reduces anxiety, headache, and insomnia
- Helps to treat high blood pressure

Caution
- Back issues

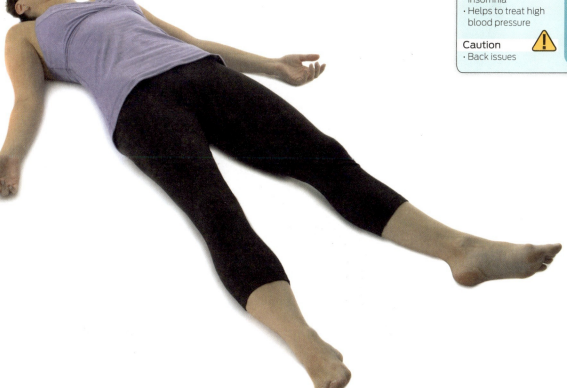

ANATOMY OF FITNESS • YOGA

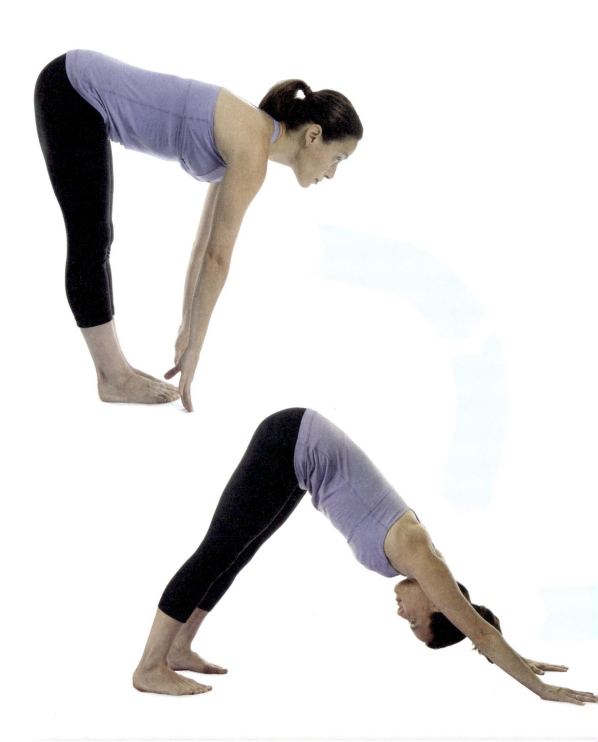

Yoga Flows

Contents

Sun Salutation A	174
Sun Salutation B	174
Hip-Opening Flow	176
Well-Rounded Flow	176
Hamstrings Flow	178
Twisting Flow	178
Intermediate Flow	180
Advanced Flow	180

Now that you have learned how to properly perform a wide range of yoga poses, it is time to start putting them together. The following yoga flows include two Sun Salutations, followed by six sequences designed to suit different needs and varying in intensity. When carrying out Sun Salutations A and B, you will find that some poses are repeated; make sure that you perform them first on one side, and then the other. If you let your breath guide you through these flows, you will find them all the more energizing, restorative, and effective for shaping your body as well as focusing your mind.

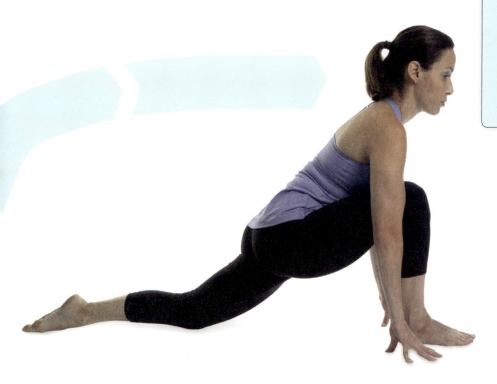

ANATOMY OF FITNESS • YOGA

Sun Salutation A

Sun Salutation A can be performed 2 to 5 times to build heat.

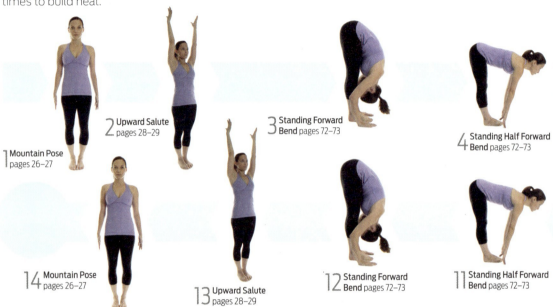

Sun Salutation B

Sun Salutation B can be performed 2 to 5 times to build heat.

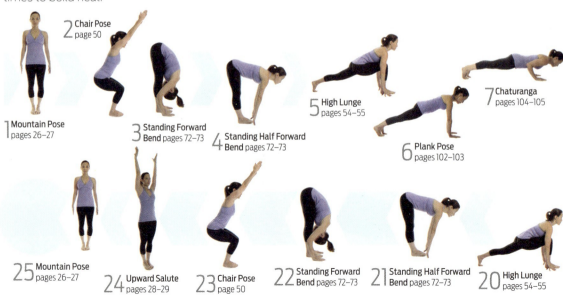

SUN SALUTATIONS

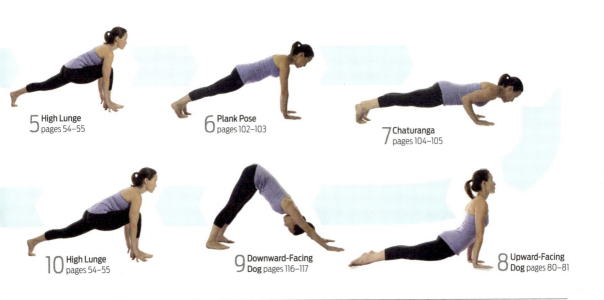

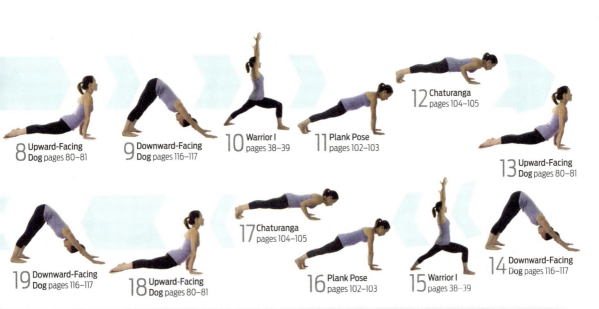

Hip-Opening Flow

Hip-Opening Flow offers an antidote to lower-body stiffness.

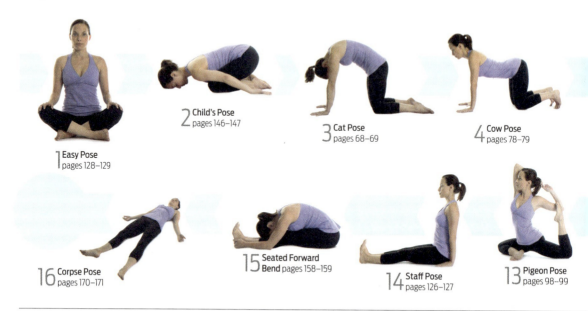

1. Easy Pose pages 128–129
2. Child's Pose pages 146–147
3. Cat Pose pages 68–69
4. Cow Pose pages 78–79
16. Corpse Pose pages 170–171
15. Seated Forward Bend pages 158–159
14. Staff Pose pages 126–127
13. Pigeon Pose pages 98–99

Well-Rounded Flow

Well-Rounded Flow has it all: balancing poses combined with hip-openers, backbends, and an inversion.

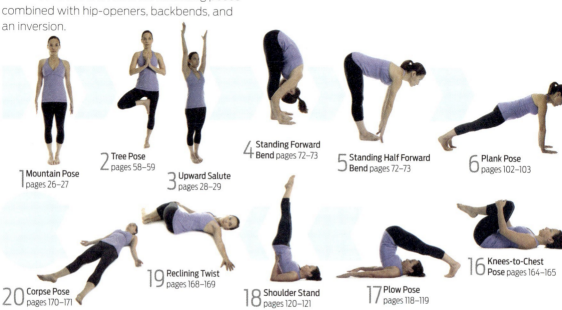

1. Mountain Pose pages 26–27
2. Tree Pose pages 58–59
3. Upward Salute pages 28–29
4. Standing Forward Bend pages 72–73
5. Standing Half Forward Bend pages 72–73
6. Plank Pose pages 102–103
20. Corpse Pose pages 170–171
19. Reclining Twist pages 168–169
18. Shoulder Stand pages 120–121
17. Plow Pose pages 118–119
16. Knees-to-Chest Pose pages 164–165

YOGA FLOWS

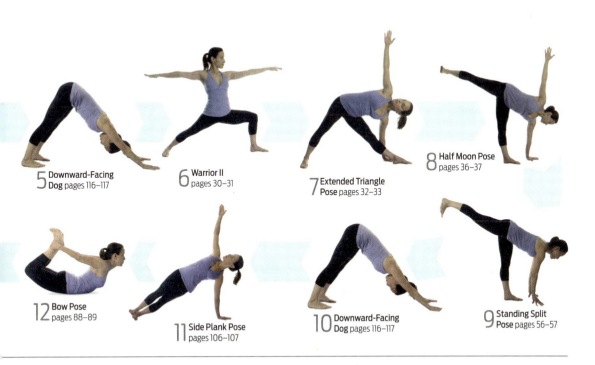

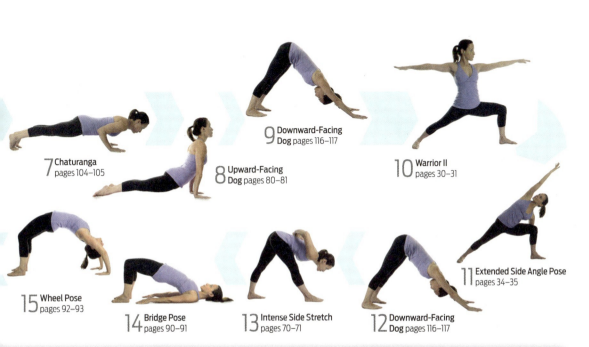

Hamstrings Flow

Hamstrings Flow gives your legs some TLC, including hamstrings stretches and internally rotated positions.

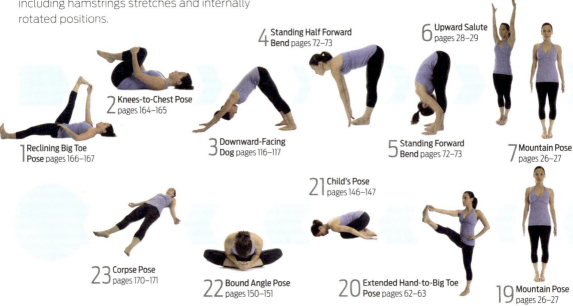

1. Reclining Big Toe Pose pages 166–167
2. Knees-to-Chest Pose pages 164–165
3. Downward-Facing Dog pages 116–117
4. Standing Half Forward Bend pages 72–73
5. Standing Forward Bend pages 72–73
6. Upward Salute pages 28–29
7. Mountain Pose pages 26–27
19. Mountain Pose pages 26–27
20. Extended Hand-to-Big Toe Pose pages 62–63
21. Child's Pose pages 146–147
22. Bound Angle Pose pages 150–151
23. Corpse Pose pages 170–171

Twisting Flow

Twisting stimulates circulation and may have a detoxifying effect. This Twisting Flow will also improve the range of motion in your spine.

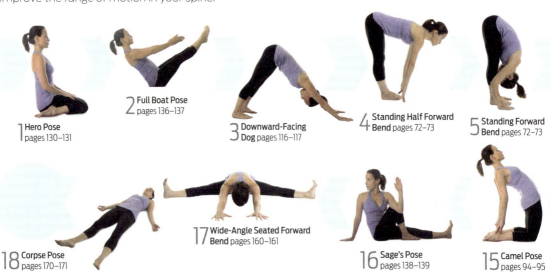

1. Hero Pose pages 130–131
2. Full Boat Pose pages 136–137
3. Downward-Facing Dog pages 116–117
4. Standing Half Forward Bend pages 72–73
5. Standing Forward Bend pages 72–73
15. Camel Pose pages 94–95
16. Sage's Pose pages 138–139
17. Wide-Angle Seated Forward Bend pages 160–161
18. Corpse Pose pages 170–171

YOGA FLOWS

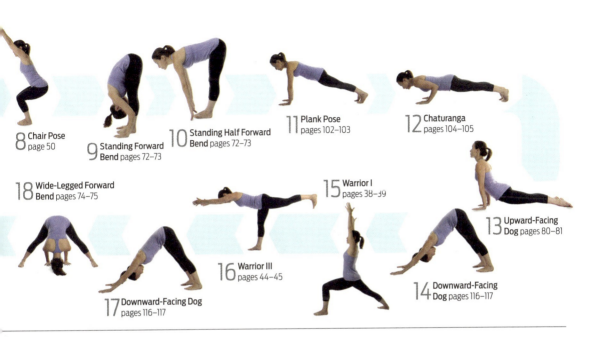

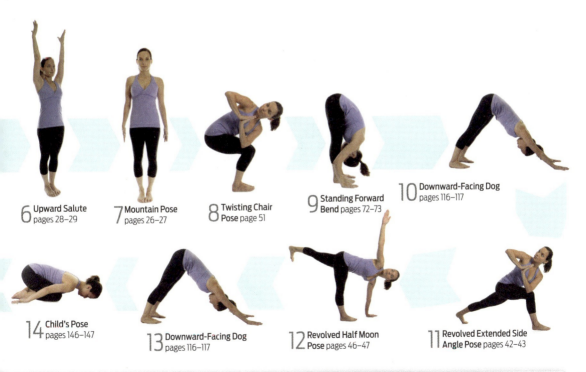

ANATOMY OF FITNESS • YOGA

Intermediate Flow

Once you've achieved basic familiarity with the practice of yoga, try this Intermediate Flow.

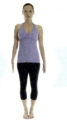
1 Mountain Pose
pages 26–27

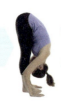
2 Standing Forward Bend pages 72–73

3 Standing Half Forward Bend pages 72–73

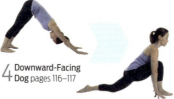
4 Downward-Facing Dog pages 116–117

5 Low Lunge
pages 52–53

6 Downward-Facing Dog pages 116–117

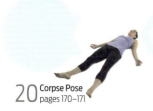
20 Corpse Pose
pages 170–171

19 Seated Forward Bend pages 158–159

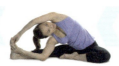
18 Revolved Head-to-Knee Pose pages 156–157

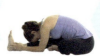
17 Head-to-Knee Forward Bend pages 154–155

16 Half Lord of the Fishes Pose pages 140–141

Advanced Flow

To make this Advanced Flow even more intense, try staying in the poses just a few breaths longer than you think you can.

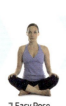
1 Easy Pose
pages 128–129

2 Downward-Facing Dog pages 116–117

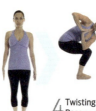
3 Mountain Pose
pages 26–27

4 Twisting Chair Pose page 51

5 Standing Forward Bend pages 72–73

6 Standing Half Forward Bend pages 72–73

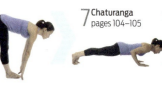
7 Chaturanga
pages 104–105

21 Fire Log Pose
pages 152–153

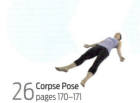
26 Corpse Pose
pages 170–171

25 Child's Pose
pages 146–147

24 Head Stand
pages 122–123

23 Dolphin Pose
(part of Head Stand) page 122

22 Bound Angle Pose
pages 150–151

YOGA FLOWS

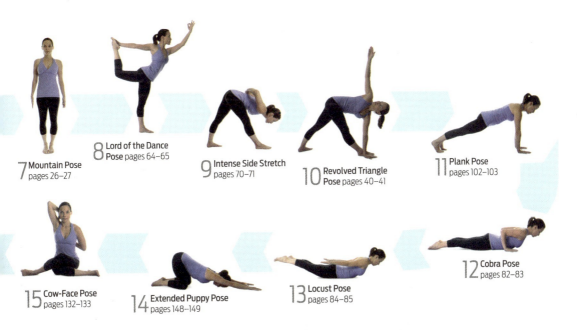

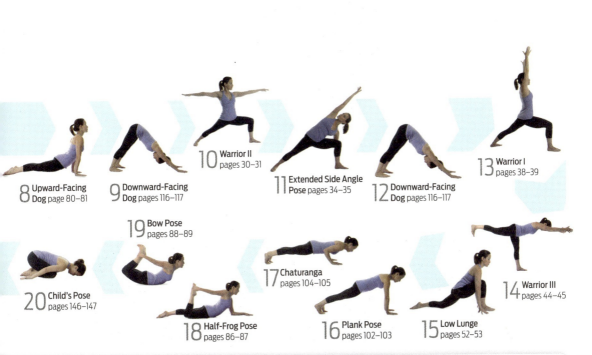

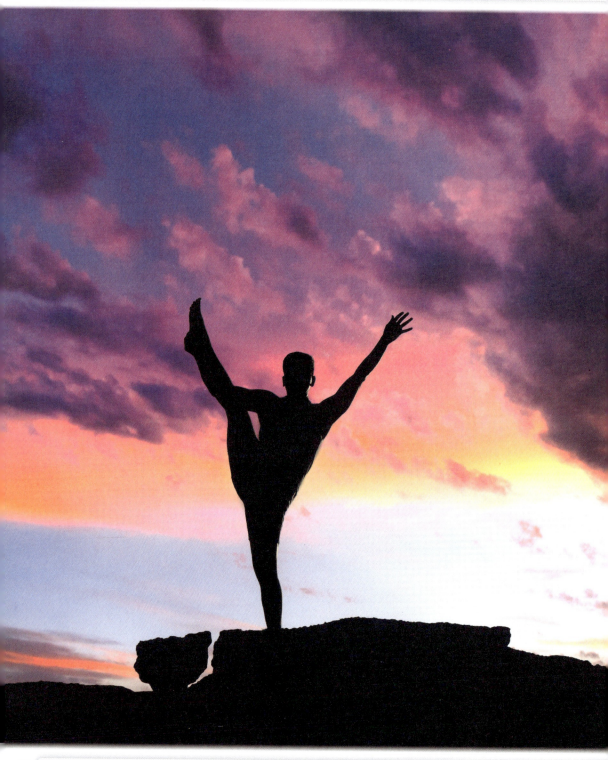

Conclusion

Congratulations on finishing *Anatomy of Fitness: Yoga*, but you are not at the end of your journey—you are just at its beginning! You now have all of the tools you need to start exploring yoga on your own. With this complete guide to yoga postures and breathing techniques, you can feel comfortable practicing at home or taking a class at a studio.

Yoga is an ongoing practice that is physical, mental, and spiritual. Create a yoga regime that fits your particular needs, which may change daily. You may find that you like a certain style of yoga or that a certain yoga teacher resonates with you, so take the time to find what works best for you.

Listen to your body, and honor where you are in the present moment, knowing that yoga is a personal journey and not a competition with yourself or those surrounding you.

As you continue, you will find that your yoga practice will seep into your life off the mat. You will build more awareness of yourself and those around you and find that you are more present in each moment. There is always time to pause and breathe.

Namaste!

Glossary

GENERAL TERMINOLOGY

abduction: Movement away from the body.

adduction: Movement toward the body.

alignment: In the yoga practice each pose has an ideal position of the body. If the body is in alignment, then it is placed in a proper way so that the muscles can work more effectively; they don't have to grip or struggle to hold the position, thus preventing injury. Each pose has its own alignment points, such as where to place the hands, feet, or torso, so learning a pose means also learning its proper points of alignment.

anterior: Located in the front.

cardiovascular exercise: Any exercise that increases the heart rate, making oxygen and nutrient-rich blood available to working muscles.

cardiovascular system: The circulatory system that distributes blood throughout the body, which includes the heart, lungs, arteries, veins, and capillaries.

cervical spine: The upper area of the spine immediately below the skull.

cool-down: A yoga pose performed at the end of the session that works to cool and relax the body after more vigorous exertion.

core: Refers to the deep muscle layers that lie close to the spine and provide structural support for the entire body. The core is divisible into two groups: major core and minor core muscles. The major muscles reside on the trunk and include the belly area and the mid and lower back. This area encompasses the pelvic floor muscles (levator ani, pubococcygeus, iliococcygeus, pubo-rectalis, and coccygeus), the abdominals (rectus abdominis, transversus abdominis, obliquus externus, and obliquus internus), the spinal extensors (multifidus spinae, erector spinae, splenius, longissimus thoracis, and semispinalis), and the diaphragm. The minor core muscles include the latissimus dorsi, gluteus maximus, and trapezius (upper, middle, and lower). These minor core muscles assist the major muscles when the body engages in activities or movements that require added stability.

eight limbs of yoga: The eight principles that define the discipline of yoga, which are 1) Yama (abstinence); 2) Niyama (observance); 3) Asana (posture); 4) Pranayama (breath control): 5) Pratyahara (sense withdrawal); 6) Dharana (concentration); 7) Dhyana (meditation); 8) Samadhi (contemplation, absorption, or superconscious state)

energy up: The subtle feeling of an upward lift.

extension: The act of straightening.

extensor muscle: A muscle serving to extend a body part away from the body.

external rotation: The act of moving a body part away from the center of the body.

flexion: The bending of a joint.

flexor muscle: A muscle that decreases the angle between two bones, as bending the arm at the elbow or raising the thigh toward the stomach.

ground down: To press the hands, feet, or other part of the body into the floor, reinforcing a solid foundation.

heel-to-arch alignment: In yoga poses, especially externally rotated postures in which the feet are separated, refers to a foot position in which the front foot is directly in front of the inner arch of the back foot.

heart-opener: In yoga, refers to a pose that stretches the hard-to-access muscles making up the chest, neck, and shoulders.

heel-to-heel alignment: In yoga poses, especially internally rotated postures in which the feet are separated, refers to the position of the feet where one is directly in front of the other.

hip-opener: A yoga pose that releases tension in hips, which is often caused by too much sitting.

iliotibial band (ITB): A thick band of fibrous tissue that runs down the outside of the leg, beginning at the hip and extending to the outer side of the tibia just below the knee joint. The band functions in concert with several of the thigh muscles to provide stability to the outside of the knee joint.

internal rotation: The act of moving a body part toward the center of the body.

lateral: Located on, or extending toward, the outside.

lumbar spine: The lower part of the spine.

GLOSSARY

medial: Located on, or extending toward, the middle.

neutral: In yoga, describes the position of the legs, pelvis, hips, or other part of the body that is neither arched nor curved forward.

neutral position (spine): A spinal position resembling an S shape when viewed in profile.

posterior: Located behind.

rotator muscle: One of a group of muscles that assist the rotation of a joint, such as the hip or the shoulder.

scapula: The protrusion of bone on the mid to upper back, also known as the "shoulder blade."

thoracic spine: The middle part of the spine warm-up: Any form of light exercise of short duration that prepares the body for more intense exercises.

yogic toe hold: A way of grasping the big toe with one hand, as called for in certain yoga poses, by placing the first two fingers under the toe and the thumb on top.

SANSKRIT TERMINOLOGY

The following glossary list explains the Sanskrit frequently used in this book.

asana: A yoga pose, posture; also the third of the eight limbs of yoga.

Anuloma Viloma: An alternate-nostril breathing technique thought to purify the energetic channels of the body in preparation for meditation. From *anuloma viloma,* "up and down," "alternate," or "reversed."

Kapalabhati: A sinus-cleansing breathing technique involving a sharp exhalation while pumping the stomach in and out. From kapal, "*skull*," and bhati, "*shining.*"

mudra: Hand position; in yoga, the positioning of the hands is thought to channel energy in specific ways.

Pranayama: The yoga science of breath control; also the fourth of the eight limbs of yoga.

Ujjayi Pranayama: A breathing technique in which the throat is slightly constricted as one inhales and exhales. From *ujjayi,* "victorious," *prana,* "life-force energy," and *ayama,* "to control or extend." This technique is also known as Victorious Breath.

Sithali: An open-mouthed breathing technique that calls for inhaling through a curled tongue.

vinyasa: A sequence or flow of breath-synchronized movements.

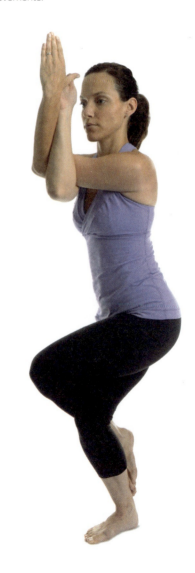

ANATOMY OF FITNESS • YOGA

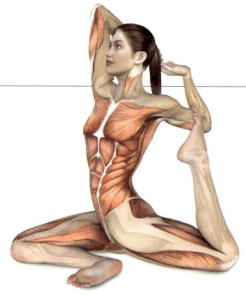

LATIN TERMINOLOGY

The following glossary list explains the Latin terminology used to describe the body's musculature. In some instance, certain words are derived from Greek, which is therein indicated.

Chest

coracobrachialis: Greek *korakoeidés*, "ravenlike," and *brachium*, "arm"

pectoralis (major and minor): *pectus*, "breast"

Abdomen

obliquus externus: *obliquus*, "slanting," and *externus*, "outward"

obliquus internus: *obliquus*, "slanting," and *internus*, "within"

rectus abdominis: *rego*, "straight, upright," and *abdomen*, "belly"

serratus anterior: *serra*, "saw," and *ante*, "before"

transversus abdominis: *transversus*, "athwart," and *abdomen*, "belly"

Neck

scalenus: Greek *skalénós*, "unequal"

semispinalis: *semi*, "half," and *spinae*, "spine"

splenius: Greek *splénion*, "plaster, patch"

sternocleidomastoideus: Greek *stérnon*, "chest," Greek *kleís*, "key," and Greek *mastoeidés*, "breastlike"

Back

erector spinae: *erectus*, "straight," and *spina*, "thorn"

latissimus dorsi: *latus*, "wide," and *dorsum*, "back"

multifidus spinae: *multifid*, "to cut into divisions," and *spinae*, "spine"

quadratus lumborum: *quadratus*, "square, rectangular," and *lumbus*, "loin"

rhomboideus: Greek *rhembesthai*, "to spin"

trapezius: Greek *trapezion*, "small table"

Shoulders

deltoideus (anterior, medial, and posterior): Greek *deltoeidés*, "delta-shaped"

infraspinatus: *infra*, "under," and *spina*, "thorn"

levator scapulae: *levare*, "to raise," and *scapulae*, "shoulder [blades]"

subscapularis: *sub*, "below," and *scapulae*, "shoulder [blades]"

supraspinatus: *supra*, "above," and *spina*, "thorn"

teres (major and minor): *teres*, "rounded"

Upper arm

biceps brachii: *biceps*, "two-headed," and *brachium*, "arm"

brachialis: *brachium*, "arm"

triceps brachii: *triceps*, "three-headed," and *brachium*, "arm"

Lower arm

anconeus: Greek *anconad*, "elbow"

brachioradialis: *brachium*, "arm," and *radius*, "spoke"

extensor carpi radialis: *extendere*, "to extend," Greek *karpós*, "wrist," and *radius*, "spoke"

extensor digitorum: *extendere*, "to extend," and *digitus*, "finger, toe"

flexor carpi pollicis longus: *flectere*, "to bend," Greek *karpós*, "wrist," *pollicis*, "thumb," and *longus*, "long"

flexor carpi radialis: *flectere*, "to bend," Greek *karpós*, "wrist," and *radius*, "spoke"

flexor carpi ulnaris: *flectere*, "to bend," Greek *karpós*, "wrist," and *ulnaris*, "forearm"

flexor digitorum: *flectere*, "to bend," and *digitus*, "finger, toe"

palmaris longus: *palmaris*, "palm," and *longus*, "long"

pronator teres: *pronate*, "to rotate," and *teres*, "rounded."

Hips

gemellus (inferior and superior): *geminus*, "twin"

gluteus maximus: Greek *gloutós*, "rump," and *maximus*, "largest"

gluteus medius: Greek *gloutós*, "rump," and *medialis*, "middle"

gluteus minimus: Greek *gloutós*, "rump," and *minimus*, "smallest"

iliopsoas: *ilium*, "groin," and Greek *psoa*, "groin muscle"

iliacus: *ilium*, "groin"

obturator externus: *obturare*, "to block," and *externus*, "outward"

obturator internus: *obturare*, "to block," and *internus*, "within"

pectineus: *pectin*, "comb"

piriformis: *pirum*, "pear," and *forma*, "shape"

quadratus femoris: *quadratus*, "square, rectangular," and *femur*, "thigh"

Upper leg

adductor longus: *adducere*, "to contract," and *longus*, "long"

adductor magnus: *adducere*, "to contract," and *magnus*, "major"

biceps femoris: *biceps*, "two-headed," and *femur*, "thigh"

gracilis: *gracilis*, "slim, slender"

rectus femoris: *rego*, "straight, upright," and *femur*, "thigh"

sartorius: *sarcio*, "to patch" or "to repair"

semimembranosus: *semi*, "half," and *membrum*, "limb"

semitendinosus: *semi*, "half," and *tendo*, "tendon"

tensor fasciae latae: *tenere*, "to stretch," *fasciae*, "band," and *latae*, "laid down"

vastus intermedius: *vastus*, "immense, huge," and *intermedius*, "between"

vastus lateralis: *vastus*, "immense, huge," and *lateralis*, "side"

vastus medialis: *vastus*, "immense, huge," and *medialis*, "middle"

Lower leg

adductor digiti minimi: *adducere*, "to contract," *digitus*, "finger, toe," and *minimum*, "smallest"

adductor hallucis: *adducere*, "to contract," and *hallex*, "big toe"

extensor digitorum: *extendere*, "to extend," and *digitus*, "finger, toe"

extensor hallucis: *extendere*, "to extend," and *hallex*, "big toe"

flexor digitorum: *flectere*, "to bend," and *digitus*, "finger, toe"

flexor hallucis: *flectere*, "to bend," and *hallex*, "big toe"

gastrocnemius: Greek *gastroknémía*, "calf [of the leg]"

peroneus: *peronei*, "of the fibula"

plantaris: *planta*, "the sole"

soleus: *solea*, "sandal"

tibialis anterior: *tibia*, "reed pipe," and *ante*, "before"

tibialis posterior: *tibia*, "reed pipe," and *posterus*, "coming after"

Icon Index

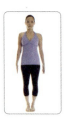
Mountain Pose
page 26

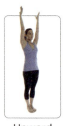
Upward Salute
page 28

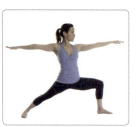
Warrior II
page 30

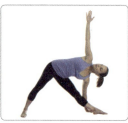
Extended Triangle Pose
page 32

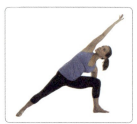
Extended Side Angle Pose
page 34

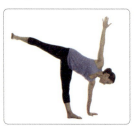
Half Moon Pose
page 36

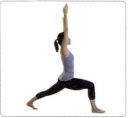
Warrior I
page 38

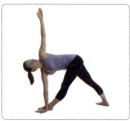
Revolved Triangle Pose
page 40

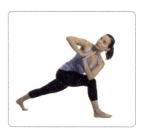
Revolved Ext. Side Angle
page 42

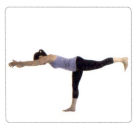
Warrior III
page 44

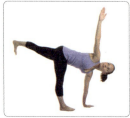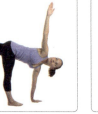
Revolved Half Moon Pose
page 46

Garland Pose
page 48

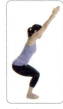
Chair Pose
page 50

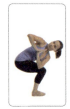
Twisting Chair Pose
page 51

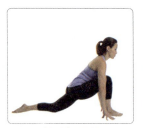
Low Lunge
page 52

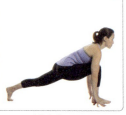
High Lunge
page 54

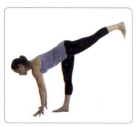
Standing Split Pose
page 56

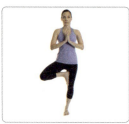
Tree Pose
page 58

ICON INDEX

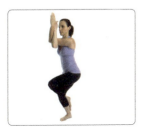
Eagle Pose
page 60

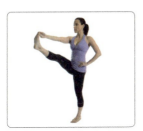
Ext. Hand-to-Big-Toe Pose
page 62

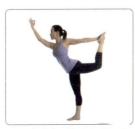
Lord of the Dance Pose
page 64

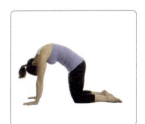
Cat Pose
page 68

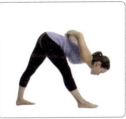
Intense Side Stretch
page 70

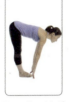
Standing Half Forward Bend
page 72

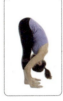
Standing Forward Bend
page 72

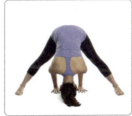
Wide-Legged Forward Bend
page 74

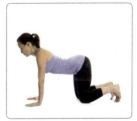
Cow Pose
page 78

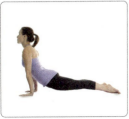
Upward-Facing Dog
page 80

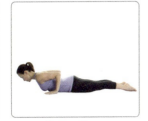
Cobra Pose
page 82

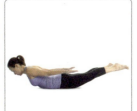
Locust Pose
page 84

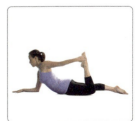
Half-Frog Pose
page 86

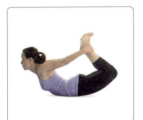
Bow Pose
page 88

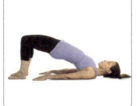
Bridge Pose
page 90

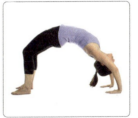
Wheel Pose
page 92

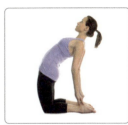
Camel Pose
page 94

ANATOMY OF FITNESS • YOGA

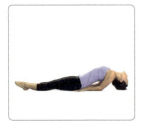
Fish Pose
page 96

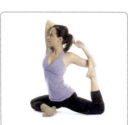
Pigeon Pose
page 98

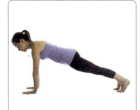
Plank Pose
page 102

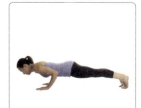
Chaturanga
page 104

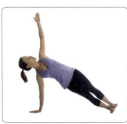
Side Plank Pose
page 106

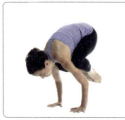
Crow Pose
page 108

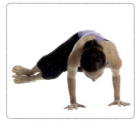
Side Crow Pose
page 110

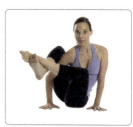
Eight-Angle Pose
page 112

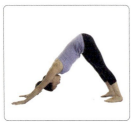
Downward-Facing Dog
page 116

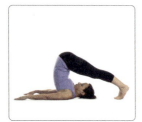
Plow Pose
page 118

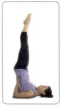
Shoulder Stand
page 120

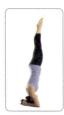
Head Stand
page 122

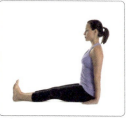
Staff Pose
page 126

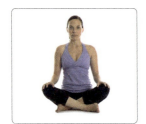
Easy Pose
page 128

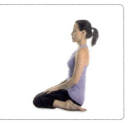
Hero Pose
page 130

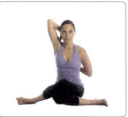
Cow-Face Pose
page 132

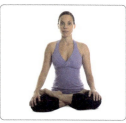
Full Lotus Pose
page 134

ICON INDEX

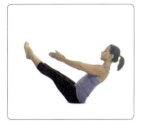
Full Boat Pose
page 136

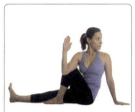
Sage's Pose
page 138

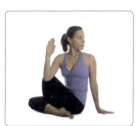
Half Lord of the
Fishes Pose page 140

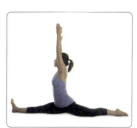
Monkey Pose
page 142

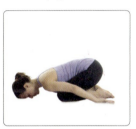
Child's Pose
page 146

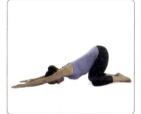
Extended Puppy Pose
page 148

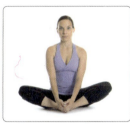
Bound Angle Pose
page 150

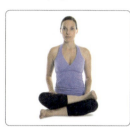
Fire Log Pose
page 152

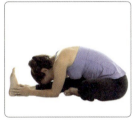
Head-to-Knee Forward Bend
page 154

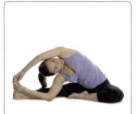
Revolved Head-to-
Knee Pose page 156

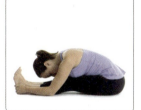
Seated Forward Bend
page 158

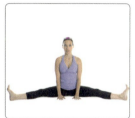
Wide-Angle Seated
Forward Bend page 160

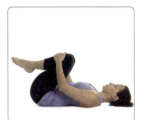
Knees-to-Chest Pose
page 164

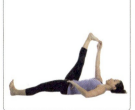
Reclining Big Toe Pose
page 166

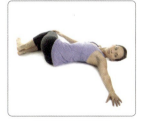
Reclining Twist
page 168

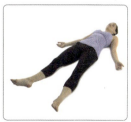
Corpse Pose
page 170

About the author

Goldie Karpel Oren began ballet training at the age of three and continued training through high school. During high school she performed with Dances Patrelle in New York as well as Ballet Rox in Boston. She received a B.A from Johns Hopkins University, Baltimore, in 2006, with a major in creative writing. After graduating from college she was a soloist with the Atlantic City Ballet.

In spring 2008, Goldie developed an injury that forced her to stop dancing but led her to yoga, which became another passion. Goldie studied yoga and became RYT certified. She now teaches yoga at several studios and works individually with private clients in their homes in New York City.

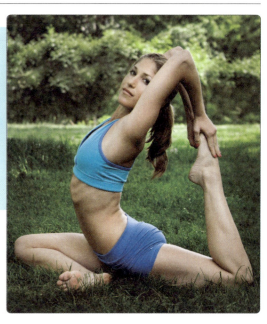

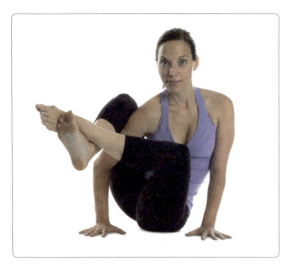

Yoga model Lana Russo is a 500-hour registered yoga teacher with the Yoga Alliance. She earned her training through the Long Island Yoga School in New York and is currently a teacher trainer there, helping others on their journey toward teaching yoga. Lana teaches at many studios throughout the Long Island area and is a current yoga ambassador for Lululemon Athletica. As a former ballet dancer, she enjoys the flow of vinyasa yoga and loves to help bring students to their own personal edge. In her spare time, she enjoys being with her husband and daughter.

Credits

All photographs by Jonathan Conklin Photography, Inc., except the following:

Page 8 middle byheaven/Shutterstock.com; page 9 middle Crepesoles/Shutterstock.com; page 10 left Ekaterina Garyuk/Shutterstock.com; page 10 bottom StockLite/Shutterstock.com; page 11 left Brooke Becker/Shutterstock.com; page 11 top right Lynn Watson/Shutterstock.com; page 11 bottom right iofoto/Shutterstock.com; page 13 insets Ajay Bhaskar/Shutterstock.com; page 15 Tom Wang/Shutterstock.com; page 18 left Dionisvera/Shutterstock.com; page 18 right rj lerich/Shutterstock.com; page 18 bottom Beth Van Trees/Shutterstock.com; page 19 left fotohunter/Shutterstock.com; page 18 top right photosync/Shutterstock.com; page 19 bottom right Zoom Team/Shutterstock.com; page 20 left Valentyn Volkov/Shutterstock.com; page 20 middle gresei/Shutterstock.com; page 20 bottom Zoom Team/Shutterstock.com; page 21 left caldix/Shutterstock.com; page 21 top right ronfromyork/Shutterstock.com; page 21 bottom right Yuri Arcurs/Shutterstock.com; pages 182–183 byheaven/Shutterstock.com.

All anatomical illustrations by Hector Aiza/3D Labz Animation India, except the following:

Small insets and full-body anatomy pages 22–23 by Linda Bucklin/Shutterstock.com and page 8 bottom by Nikitina Olga/Shutterstock.com.